Psychological Issues for the Oral and Maxillofacial Surgeon

Guest Editor

HILLEL EPHROS, DMD, MD

ORAL AND MAXILLOFACIAL SURGERY CLINICS OF NORTH AMERICA

www.oralmaxsurgery.theclinics.com

Consulting Editor
RICHARD H. HAUG, DDS

November 2010 • Volume 22 • Number 4

SAUNDERS an imprint of ELSEVIER, Inc.

W.B. SAUNDERS COMPANY
A Division of Elsevier Inc.

1600 John F. Kennedy Blvd. ● Suite 1800 ● Philadelphia, PA 19103-2899

www.oralmaxsurgery.theclinics.com

ORAL AND MAXILLOFACIAL SURGERY CLINICS OF NORTH AMERICA Volume 22, Number 4
November 2010 ISSN 1042-3699, ISBN-13: 978-1-4377-2473-8

Editor: John Vassallo; j.vassallo@elsevier.com
Developmental Editor: Donald Mumford

Oral and Maxillofacial Surgery Clinics of North America (ISSN 1042-3699) is published quarterly by Elsevier Inc., 360 Park Avenue South, New York, NY 10010-1710. Months of issue are February, May, August, and November. Business and Editorial Offices: 1600 John F. Kennedy Blvd., Suite 1800, Philadelphia, PA 19103-2899. Periodicals postage paid at New York, NY and additional mailing offices. Subscription prices are $329.00 per year for US individuals, $490.00 per year for US institutions, $147.00 per year for US students and residents, $383.00 per year for Canadian individuals, $583.00 per year for Canadian institutions, $441.00 per year for international individuals, $583.00 per year for international institutions and $200.00 per year for Canadian and foreign students/residents. To receive student/resident rate, orders must be accompanied by name or affiliated institution, date of term, and the *signature* of program/residency coordinator on institution letterhead. Orders will be billed at individual rate until proof of status is received. Foreign air speed delivery is included in all *Clinics* subscription prices. All prices are subject to change without notice. **POSTMASTER:** Send address changes to *Oral and Maxillofacial Surgery Clinics of North America,* Elsevier Periodicals Customer Service, 11830 Westline Industrial Drive, St. Louis, MO 63146. Tel: 1-800-654-2452 (U.S. and Canada); 314-447-8871 (outside U.S. and Canada). Fax: 314-447-8029. E-mail: journalscustomerservice-usa@elsevier.com (for print support); journalsonlinesupport-usa@elsevier.com (for online support).

Reprints. For copies of 100 or more, of articles in this publication, please contact the Commercial Reprints Department, Elsevier Inc., 360 Park Avenue South, New York, NY 10010-1710. Tel.: 212-633-3812; Fax: 212-462-1935; Email: reprints@elsevier.com.

Oral and Maxillofacial Surgery Clinics of North America is covered in MEDLINE/PubMed (*Index Medicus*).

Printed and bound in the United Kingdom
Transferred to Digital Print 2011

Contributors

CONSULTING EDITOR

RICHARD H. HAUG, DDS
Carolinas Center for Oral Health
Charlotte, North Carolina

GUEST EDITOR

HILLEL EPHROS, DMD, MD
Professor and Chairman, Dentistry and
Oral and Maxillofacial Surgery, Seton Hall
University School of Health and Medical
Sciences, South Orange; Oral and
Maxillofacial Surgery Program Director and
Chairman, Department of Dentistry,
St Joseph's Regional Medical Center;
Medical Director, The Regional Craniofacial
Center, St Joseph's Children's Hospital,
Paterson, New Jersey

AUTHORS

MEREDITH BLITZ, DDS
Assistant Professor, Division of Dentistry,
Department of Oral and Maxillofacial Surgery,
Seton Hall University, South Orange; University
of Medicine and Dentistry of New Jersey,
Newark; Staff Oral and Maxillofacial Surgeon,
Department of Oral and Maxillofacial Surgery,
St Joseph's Regional Medical Center,
Paterson, New Jersey

RACHEL BLUEBOND-LANGNER, MD
Division of Plastic and Reconstructive Surgery,
Johns Hopkins School of Medicine, Baltimore,
Maryland

SCOTT BOLDING, DDS
Oral and Maxillofacial Surgeon, Private
Practice; Chief Executive Officer, U.S.
HealthRecord, Fayetteville, Arkansas

KATE CERINO BRITTON, MSEd, MA, BCBA
Principal, Alpine Learning Group, Paramus,
New Jersey

JENEV CADDELL, PsyD
Private Practice, New York, New York

CANICE E. CRERAND, PhD
Division of Plastic and Reconstructive
Surgery, Department of Psychology,
The Edwin and Fannie Gray Hall Center for
Human Appearance, The Children's Hospital
of Philadelphia, Philadelphia, Pennsylvania

RENIE DANIEL, DMD, MS
Resident, Department of Oral and Maxillofacial
Surgery, St Joseph's Regional Medical Center,
Paterson, New Jersey

ROBERT J. DEFALCO, DDS
Staff Oral and Maxillofacial Surgeon,
Attending Physician, St Joseph's Regional
Medical Center, Department of Oral and
Maxillofacial Surgery, Paterson; Clinical
Assistant Professor, Seton Hall University
School of Health and Medical Sciences,
South Orange, New Jersey

HILLEL EPHROS, DMD, MD
Professor and Chairman, Dentistry and Oral
and Maxillofacial Surgery, Seton Hall University
School of Health and Medical Sciences, South
Orange; Oral and Maxillofacial Surgery
Program Director and Chairman, Department
of Dentistry, St Joseph's Regional Medical
Center; Medical Director, The Regional
Craniofacial Center, St Joseph's Children's
Hospital, Paterson, New Jersey

MICHAEL ERLICHMAN, DDS
Staff Oral and Maxillofacial Surgeon,
St Joseph's Regional Medical Center,
Department of Oral and Maxillofacial Surgery,
Paterson; Clinical Associate Professor, Seton
Hall University School of Health and Medical
Sciences, South Orange, New Jersey

**MARCELLA FRANK, DO, FCCP, FACOI,
DABSM**
Co-Medical Director, The Center for Sleep
Medicine, Capital Health's Center for Sleep
Medicine, Trenton, New Jersey

PAUL E. GATES, DDS, MBA
Chair, Department of Dentistry, Bronx Lebanon
Hospital Center; Chair, Dr Martin Luther King
Jr, Community Health Center, Bronx,
New York, New York

MATTHEW R. HLAVACEK, MD, DDS
Clinical Assistant Professor, Departments of
Surgery and Oral and Maxillofacial Surgery,
University of Missouri-Kansas City, Schools of
Medicine and Dentistry; Attending Staff, Facial
and Cosmetic Surgery, St Luke's Hospital,
Kansas City, Missouri

NANCY JUST, PhD, ABPP
Fellow, American Academy of Clinical
Psychology; Diplomate in Clinical Psychology,
American Board of Professional Psychology;
Director, Advanced Psychological Specialists,
Ridgewood, New Jersey

HARRIET S. LANGLEY, MD
Chief of Nephrology, Menorah Medical Center,
Overland Park; Clinical Assistant Professor
of Medicine, University of Missouri-Kansas City
of Medicine, Kansas, Missouri

LAUREN D. LAPORTA, MD, DFAPA
Chairman, Department of Psychiatry,
St Joseph's Healthcare System, Paterson,
New Jersey; Assistant Clinical Professor,
Mt Sinai School of Medicine, New York,
New York; Clinical Assistant Professor,
Department of Medicine, Seton Hall University
School of Health and Medical Sciences,
South Orange; Clinical Assistant Professor,
Department of Psychiatry, University of
Medicine and Dentistry of New Jersey-New
Jersey Medical School, Newark, New Jersey;
Associate Professor, Department of
Psychiatry, St George's University, University
Center, Grenada, West Indies

JENNIFER LYNE, MA
PhD Candidate, Clinical Psychology Program,
Fairleigh Dickinson University, Teaneck,
New Jersey; Research Associate,
Interpersonal Communications Laboratory,
Department of Communication Sciences, Child
Psychiatry, Psychiatric Institute, New York,
New York

FARIDEH M. MADANI, DMD
Professor, Department of Oral Medicine,
Robert Schattner Center, University of
Pennsylvania, School of Dental Medicine,
Philadelphia, Pennsylvania

MANSOOR MADANI, DMD, MD
Chairman, Department of Oral and
Maxillofacial Surgery, Capital Health Regional
Medical Center, Trenton, New Jersey;
Associate Professor, Oral and Maxillofacial
Surgery, Temple University, Philadelphia;
Director, Bala Institute of Oral and Facial
Surgery, Bala Cynwyd, Pennsylvania

LEANNE MAGEE, PhD
Division of Plastic and Reconstructive Surgery,
Department of Psychology, The Edwin and
Fannie Gray Hall Center for Human
Appearance, The Children's Hospital of
Philadelphia, Philadelphia, Pennsylvania

JOHN J. MITCHELL Jr, PhD
Chair, Department of Biomedical Ethics,
School of Health and Medical Sciences;
Seton Hall University, South Orange,
New Jersey

STEVEN D. PASSIK, PhD
Associate Attending Psychologist,
Department of Psychiatry and Behavioral
Sciences, Memorial Sloan-Kettering Cancer
Center; Associate Professor, Department
of Psychiatry, Weill-Cornell Medical Center,
New York, New York

STEVEN J. PRSTOJEVICH, MD, DDS, FACS
Medical Director, Facial and Cosmetic
Surgery, St Luke's Hospital; Clinical
Associate Professor, Department of Oral
and Maxillofacial Surgery, University of
Missouri-Kansas City, Schools of Medicine
and Dentistry; Associate Program Director,
Oral and Maxillofacial Surgery, University
of Missouri-Kansas City, St Luke's Hospital,
Kansas City, Missouri

WALTER F. RICCI, MD
Clinical Professor, Department of Psychiatry,
University of Missouri-Kansas City, School
of Medicine; Training and Supervising
Psychoanalyst, Greater Kansas City
Psychoanalytic Institute, Kansas City,
Missouri

EDUARDO D. RODRIGUEZ, MD, DDS
Division of Plastic and Reconstructive Surgery,
R Adams Cowley Shock Trauma Center and
the University of Maryland Medical Systems,
Baltimore, Maryland

DAVID S. ROSEN, MD, MPH
Professor, Departments of Pediatrics and
Communicable Disease, Internal Medicine
and Psychiatry, University of Michigan
Medical School; Chief, Section of Teenage
and Young Adult Health, Division of Child
Behavioral Health, Department of Pediatrics,
University of Michigan Health System,
Ann Arbor, Michigan

DAVID B. SARWER, PhD
Associate Professor of Psychology in
Psychiatry and Surgery, Division of Plastic
Surgery, Department of Surgery, The Edwin
and Fannie Gray Hall Center for Human
Appearance; Department of Psychiatry,
Center for Weight and Eating Disorders,
The University of Pennsylvania School
of Medicine, Philadelphia, Pennyslyvania

PAUL M. SZUMITA, PharmD, BCPS
Clinical Pharmacy Practice Manager,
Department of Pharmacy Services, Brigham
and Women's Hospital, Pharmacy
Administration; Adjunct Assistant Professor of
Pharmacy, Critical Care, Northeastern
University Bouvé College of Pharmacy and
Health Sciences, Boston, Massachusetts;
Adjunct Assistant Professor of Pharmacy,
Critical Care, University of Rhode Island,
College of Pharmacy, Kingston, Rhode Island

RICHARD P. SZUMITA, DDS
Associate Program Director, Oral and
Maxillofacial Surgery Residency Training
Program; Associate Chairman, Department
of Dentistry, St Joseph's Regional Medical
Center, Paterson; Associate Clinical Professor,
Department of Dentistry and Oral and
Maxillofacial Surgery, School of Health and
Medical Sciences, Seton Hall University, South
Orange; Private Practice, Paramus and
Little Falls, New Jersey

SHARANG TICKOO
Research Assistant, Department of
Psychiatry and Behavioral Sciences,
Memorial Sloan-Kettering Cancer Center,
New York, New York

ALBERT W. WU, MD, MPH
Department of Health Policy and Management,
Johns Hopkins Bloomberg School of Public
Health, Baltimore, Maryland

Contents

The Need for Preoperative Psychological Risk Assessment　　　　431

Jennifer Lyne, Hillel Ephros, and Scott Bolding

Adverse psychological outcomes are more prevalent among patients undergoing elective, appearance-altering surgery than are physical complications. Patients may experience depression, posttraumatic stress disorder, or an exacerbation of preexisting symptoms related to body dysmorphic disorder. Some have directed anger against themselves or against the operating surgeon with suicide, litigation, harassment, and homicide, all well documented. Although there are well-established protocols to conduct medical and anesthetic risk stratification, such protocols do not exist for psychological risk assessment (PRA). The literature related to this is reviewed, the need for PRA is discussed, and an approach to PRA for dentists and surgeons is proposed.

Psychological Risks Associated with Appearance-Altering Procedures: Issues "Facing" Cosmetic Surgery　　　　439

Walter F. Ricci, Steven J. Prstojevich, Harriet S. Langley, and Matthew R. Hlavacek

There is a dynamic and fluid relationship between cosmetic surgery and psychology that requires careful and constant attention from the surgeon. Surgeons all desire a "short and sweet" checklist evaluation that tells them if it is safe for the patient to undergo an elective surgical procedure. Obviously, this is wishful thinking. It is asking too much for surgeons to be able to quantify the overall psychological risk. Rather, they should objectively screen, review, and evaluate as many of the variables as possible. These include but are not limited to the surgical issue, the personality of the patient, the patient's family and/or relationships, and the overall context of the situation. Surgeons should also reflect on both their technical expertise and limitations and the patient's personal resiliency.

Body Dysmorphic Disorder in Patients Who Seek Appearance-Enhancing Medical Treatments　　　　445

David B. Sarwer, Canice E. Crerand, and Leanne Magee

Most patients who seek appearance-enhancing medical treatments report some degree of body image dissatisfaction, which is believed to motivate the pursuit of these treatments. However, patients with extreme body image dissatisfaction may be suffering from a psychiatric disorder known as body dysmorphic disorder (BDD). This article reviews BDD, including its clinical features and prevalence in medical settings. Although patients with BDD frequently seek cosmetic treatments to address their appearance-related distress, such treatments are rarely beneficial. The article concludes with recommendations for patient and provider safety.

Personality Disorders in Patients Seeking Appearance-Altering Procedures　　　　455

Jenev Caddell and Jennifer Lyne

The practice of psychological risk assessment (PRA) is an indispensable component of the screening process for patients seeking elective appearance-altering procedures (AAPs). Despite the need for more literature in PRA, some risk factors for psychological adverse outcomes have been established. Among these risk factors are personality disorders. This article provides some background regarding psychological risk factors associated with personality disorders for patients seeking AAPs and a brief introduction to personality disorders for the surgeons to be better prepared to identify these conditions while conducting a PRA.

The management of a child who requires a medical procedure is a challenging issue for the oral and maxillofacial surgeon (OMS) and practitioners in the dental specialties. The office of the OMS is traditionally one in which short outpatient procedures are performed within brief appointment times often using only local anesthesia. For typical children, this brief procedure may be difficult, and for children with behavioral challenges, it may be impossible without the use of behavioral management techniques or pharmacologic modalities. Practitioners must be aware of current trends in pediatric mental health and should develop treatment protocols to avoid complications.

Complications and undesired outcomes happen to some patients of virtually all physicians, at all stages in their careers. Bad outcomes can be a consequence of disease processes, the premorbid condition of the patient, or the errors that occur in the process of health care. These errors include, but are by no means confined to, surgeon error. Regardless of the reason for the bad outcome, the surgeon is obligated to discuss the event with the patient and the family. This article reviews the benefits, barriers, and legal implications of the discussion and describes the disclosure process.

The specialty of oral and maxillofacial surgery has had at its core the foundations of anesthesia and pain and anxiety control. This article attempts to refamiliarize the reader with clinical pearls helpful in the management of patients with chronic pain conditions. The authors also hope to highlight the interplay of chronic pain and psychology as it relates to the oral and maxillofacial surgery patient. To that end, the article outlines and reviews the neurophysiology of pain, the definitions of pain, conditions encountered by the oral and maxillofacial surgeon that produce chronic pain, the psychological impact and comorbidities associated with patients experiencing chronic pain conditions, and concepts of multimodal treatment for patients experiencing chronic pain conditions.

Health professionals are subject to higher levels of stress than the average worker. Little has been written on these subjects, specifically in oral and maxillofacial surgeons. Anecdotally, dentists have been singled out as the health care professionals more likely to be subjected to severe stress, burnout, failed marriages, depression, substance abuse, and commit suicide. However, with oral and maxillofacial surgery being a particularly high-stress specialty of dentistry, a study of the dental literature regarding stress may be relevant. This article explores the myths and realities of stress and burnout in oral and maxillofacial surgeons and the coping skills, both adaptive and maladaptive used by practitioners to deal with their stress. This article also offers some practical suggestions for improving both the mental and physical health of oral and maxillofacial surgeons.

Oral and Maxillofacial Surgery Clinics of North America

FORTHCOMING ISSUES

February 2011

Reoperative Oral and Maxillofacial Surgery
Rui Fernandes, DMD, MD
and Luis Vega, DDS,
Guest Editors

May 2011

Toward Tissue Engineering in Maxillofacial Reconstruction
Ole T. Jensen, DDS, MS, *Guest Editor*

August 2011

Dento-Alveolar Complications
Dennis-Duke R. Yamashita, DDS
and James P. McAndrews, DDS,
Guest Editors

RECENT ISSUES

August 2010

Alveolar Bone Grafting Techniques for Dental Implant Preparation
Peter D. Waite, MPH, DDS, MD, *Guest Editor*

May 2010

Collaborative Care of the Facial Injury Patient
Vivek Shetty, DDS, Dr Med Dent and
Grant N. Marshall, PhD, *Guest Editors*

February 2010

Clinical Innovation and Technology in Craniomaxillofacial Surgery
Bernard J. Costello, DMD, MD, FACS,
Guest Editor

RELATED INTEREST

Facial Plastic Surgery Clinics of North America, May 2008 (Vol. 16, No. 2)
The Difficult Patient
Donn R. Chatham, MD, *Guest Editor*

THE CLINICS ARE NOW AVAILABLE ONLINE!

Access your subscription at:
www.theclinics.com

Preface
Psychological Issues for the Oral and Maxillofacial Surgeon

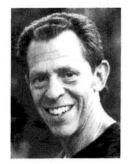

Hillel Ephros, DMD, MD
Guest Editor

"The only normal people are the ones you don't know very well."

—*Alfred Adler*

As a resident at a Veterans Administration hospital in the 1980s, I was trained to send every patient for psychological screening as part of the workup for orthognathic surgery. The protocol had been developed in response to a patient's troubling adverse psychological outcome despite a satisfactory surgical result. This outcome was not an isolated event. In fact, it has been reported that negative psychological consequences outnumber physical complications in the realm of elective, appearance-altering surgery. While we may possess good instincts and display excellent judgment, those of us who perform appearance-altering procedures and who are not mental health professionals may be inadequately prepared to conduct psychological risk assessment. Even when treatment is surgical, the therapeutic relationship plays an important role in the patient's perception of the outcome and of the perioperative experience. Many of us may feel uncomfortable when our patients are manipulative or difficult, are substance abusers, are chronic pain sufferers, or face incurable illness. Our training may not have given us the tools to recognize personality disorders or the psychological impact of fragmented sleep or to note subtleties that might lead to the diagnosis of an eating disorder. Moreover, as doctors, when stress and burnout affect us, we may be the last to acknowledge the existence of a problem.

Oral and maxillofacial surgery and psychology interface in many ways. The intent of this issue is to explore clinically relevant areas from both perspectives. I am most grateful to all of the clinicians and researchers who agreed to participate in this project. I am particularly appreciative of the open-minded contributors who took my call without ever having met me or spoken with me before and who agreed to spend hours of their time developing this material for the readers of this series.

This issue is dedicated to two men who helped to shape me personally and professionally. They are my father, Abraham Z. Ephros, and one of my principal mentors, Dr John A. Paterson, known to all as Jack.

Abraham Z. Ephros was a civil engineer who designed bridges, tunnels, and dams. He was a decorated World War II veteran who was fortunate to have earned a Purple Heart without suffering any long-term, disabling consequences of his injuries. He taught me a great deal and his approach to his work certainly had an impact on me. However, my dad's most profound effects on me relate to who he was as a human being and how he lived his life. Just like his father, who was a celebrated musician, my dad approached life with humility,

Oral Maxillofacial Surg Clin N Am 22 (2010) xi–xii
doi:10.1016/j.coms.2010.08.001
1042-3699/10/$ – see front matter © 2010 Elsevier Inc. All rights reserved.

humor, kindness, honesty, optimism, and an unparalleled ability to extract joy from each moment. His gift to me was far greater than the privilege of inheriting some of his genes. The example he set every day created a template for a life of happiness, fulfillment, and service.

Jack Paterson was a gifted surgeon, an outstanding educator, and a remarkable visionary—a larger-than-life figure whose aura was palpable and powerful. His dedication to his specialty, to his residents, and to the ethical delivery of health care was evident throughout his distinguished career. After serving as a chairman, a senior vice president for medical affairs, and a dean, he chose to step down and pursue a PhD in medical ethics. His premature passing denied him the opportunity to complete that program, but his legacy remains. Forever embedded within each of us lucky enough to have been close to Jack is a clear view of integrity, a healthy relationship with hard work, and a profound respect for knowledge.

Jack and my dad were very different people, but they both recognized and respected everyone's humanity and looked beyond the surface, trying to understand and appreciate each person they encountered. It is my hope that this issue will provide some insights into our patients and ourselves, beyond anatomy and physiology, in a realm not so familiar to surgeons.

"If the human brain were so simple that we could understand it, we would be so simple that we couldn't."
                                    —*Emerson M. Pugh*

Finally, I would like to acknowledge and thank all of my residents from whom I have learned so much, particularly those who stayed and became part of the faculty. Also, special thanks to my friends on the Board's Examination Committee as well as to Kayla, Jake, Maura, Heather, and to the many musicians with whom I share my "other" life.

Hillel Ephros, DMD, MD
St Joseph's Regional Medical Center
Department of Dentistry/Oral and Maxillofacial Surgery
703 Main Street
Paterson, NJ 07503, USA

E-mail address:
ephrosh@sjhmc.org

The Need for Preoperative Psychological Risk Assessment

Jennifer Lyne, MA[a,b], Hillel Ephros, DMD, MD[c,d,e],*,
Scott Bolding, DDS[f,g]

KEYWORDS

- Preoperative psychological risk assessment
- Adverse psychological outcomes
- Appearance-altering procedures • Elective surgery

Every clinician who performs elective surgery recognizes the need to medically evaluate patients before any procedure. This process results in risk stratification and gives the clinician an opportunity to minimize the likelihood of harm to patients by leading to one of the following conclusions:

- The procedure may take place without special considerations or modifications.
- There may be benefit to modifying the proposed treatment or somehow optimizing patients' anticipated response to the intervention.
- The procedure should be deferred until more information can be obtained through additional testing or consultation so that appropriate actions may be taken to enhance patient safety and produce the best possible outcome.
- The required level of care is not available from the provider or facility conducting the risk stratification and the process leads to an appropriate referral.

Conducting this type of medical risk assessment process is standard practice and has been the subject of various guidelines and regulations.[1–11] Procedures done using some form of anesthesia generate similar activity by the anesthesiologist who evaluates patient data and assigns a classification that reflects risk and helps to guide management. On occasion, this process may lead to the postponement of an elective procedure by the anesthesiologist. The American Society of Anesthesiologists' classification system, developed in 1941 and revised in 1984, is widely used, as are related guidelines regarding preanesthesia testing requirements based on the history, the physical findings, and the type of surgery contemplated.[10]

The primary goal of these rigorous processes is to minimize the likelihood of surgical and anesthetic complications. For patients who choose to undergo appearance-altering procedures (AAP), adverse psychological outcomes are more prevalent than physical complications.[12] Despite this, there are no established protocols for

a Clinical Psychology Program, Fairleigh Dickinson University, 1000 River Road, Teaneck, NJ 07666, USA
b Interpersonal Communications Laboratory, Department of Communication Sciences, Child Psychiatry, New York Psychiatric Institute, 1051 Riverside Drive, New York, NY 10032, USA
c Department of Dentistry and Oral and Maxillofacial Surgery, Seton Hall University School of Health and Medical Sciences, 400 South Orange Avenue, South Orange, NJ 07079, USA
d Department of Dentistry, St Joseph's Regional Medical Center, 703 Main Street, Paterson, NJ 07503, USA
e The Regional Craniofacial Center, St Joseph's Children's Hospital, 703 Main Street, Paterson, NJ 07503, USA
f Private Practice, Fayetteville, AR 72703, USA
g U.S. HealthRecord, 4058 North College Avenue, Suite 250, Fayetteville, AR 72703, USA
* Corresponding author.
E-mail address: ephrosh@sjhmc.org

Oral Maxillofacial Surg Clin N Am 22 (2010) 431–437
doi:10.1016/j.coms.2010.07.001
1042-3699/10/$ — see front matter © 2010 Elsevier Inc. All rights reserved.

psychological risk assessment (PRA) that enable clinicians performing AAP to risk stratify their patients in terms of psychological fitness. Obstacles may include the failure of standard personality inventories to consistently identify relevant psychopathology in the population in question and the limitations of subjective, interview-based assessments.[13–15] In addition, surgeons and other clinicians performing AAP may have the sense that they use clinical judgment with reasonable success when conducting informal psychological screenings. Nonetheless, the case for effective PRA is based on the prevalence of psychological adverse outcomes in the population undergoing AAP, including anecdotal reports of suicide, assault, and homicide.[12] The rationale for PRA is also built on assumptions that seem intuitively obvious, although they may lack the support of hard evidence. These assumptions include the following:

- The population seeking AAP is inherently different than the general population.
- There are psychological conditions and other factors that elevate the risk for adverse psychological outcomes in association with AAP.
- Surgeons and other clinicians who are not mental health specialists may not have adequate tools to recognize the more subtle presentations of some psychological conditions that may predispose to adverse outcomes.
- Failure to psychologically risk stratify patients seeking AAP may result in harm to patients or harm to the clinician.

The population seeking AAP is inherently different than the general population. This distinction has been reported and there is some evidence to suggest that this might be accepted as fact. Wright stated his view quite plainly: "Every esthetic surgery patient is a potential problem patient."[16] Even more aggressive was the statement by Linn and Goldman that all cosmetic surgery patients are "in effect, psychiatric patients."[17] In fact, some plastic surgeons have referred to what they do as "psychiatry with a scalpel." Two compelling, long-term studies compared AAP seekers against controls and evaluated patients years later. In a recent study, 3257 women seeking breast augmentation between 1965 and 1993 were evaluated in comparison with an untreated control group. Mental illness, manifested most notably as substance abuse and suicide, was much more prevalent in the augmented group. In fact, suicide and alcohol and drug-related deaths in the augmented group were 3 times more likely than in the control group.[18]

A much older report compared 194 individuals, all of whom had undergone rhinoplasty (118 electively and 78 because of trauma or disease). Ten years later, there were remarkable differences noted between the two groups. In the elective rhinoplasty cohort, 38% had a documented psychological disorder and 4% were schizophrenics. Among those who had rhinoplasty done because of trauma or disease, only 8% had a psychological disorder and none were diagnosed with schizophrenia.[19] The suggested relationship between psychological conditions and the desire for esthetic surgery does not imply that AAP should be withheld across the board. There is strong support for the psychological benefits of AAP, including orthognathic surgery in appropriately selected patients.[20,21] However, among those seeking AAP, there may be a significant subpopulation of individuals whose motivations, expectations, and emotional fitness are questionable.

Some psychological conditions and other factors elevate the risk for adverse outcomes with AAP. Rankin and Borah reported a strong correlation between a history of mental illness and the occurrence of postoperative psychological complications.[22] Included among the factors listed by Honingman and Phillips associated with poor psychological outcomes after AAP are personality disorders, body dysmorphic disorder (BDD), depression, and anxiety.[23] The prudent clinician might consider whether a distorted self-image is driving the need for change and whether expectations are realistic. An extensive review of the literature by Sarwer and colleagues[13] suggests that attempts to detect psychopathology in prospective patients, and to assign risk based on such diagnoses, may not serve the needs of the clinician performing AAP. In fact, some studies suggest that even at-risk patients may benefit from such procedures. In Sarwer's review, a continuum of body image dissatisfaction is described ranging from normative discontent through body dysmorphic disorder. In patients with BDD, dissatisfaction becomes pathologic and behavior is affected. Patients with an insatiable need for AAP and those who present with what the clinician views as a minimal deformity may fit into this category. Clearly, for patients with BDD, AAP is likely to lead to continued dissatisfaction, may exacerbate psychological illness, and could lead to adverse outcomes.

Subtle presentations of conditions elevating risk with AAP may not be easily detected. No studies were identified that support this assumption.

However, simply comparing the training of dentists and physicians who do not practice a mental health specialty with the education provided to those who do, it is likely that mental health specialists are better equipped to pick up subtleties and assess patients seeking AAP. For example, it is imaginable that a well-meaning surgeon treating patients who seem particularly devoted and complimentary might miss clues that would lead a trained specialist to the diagnosis of borderline personality disorder. Intelligent patients with certain personality disorders may be clever and manipulative enough to avoid being red flagged by even an experienced clinician. A detailed discussion of personality disorders by Jenev Vahe and Jennifer Lyne is found elsewhere in this issue and in the work of Shedler and Westen.[24–26]

Failure to conduct PRA may cause harm to patients or to the clinician. It is not known whether the well-documented cases of psychological adverse outcome associated with AAP might have been avoided by conducting some form of risk stratification. Nonetheless, it seems reasonable to assume that at least some of these patients might have been identified, surgery could have been withheld, and the adverse outcome potentially averted in these cases. Others might have benefited from preoperative identification leading to supportive care, counseling, or some other approach that might have mitigated the patient's response to the AAP. Frances Cooke Macgregor concludes that of the factors leading to patient dissatisfaction with technically satisfactory surgery, the "most basic one is the surgeon's initial failure to interview and carefully evaluate the patient, or to have an evaluation done by a professional skilled in the area."[27]

Based on these assumptions and a review of the literature that exists on this subject, the potential benefits of conducting PRA are clear. The potential complications associated with a failure to conduct PRA are also evident and are likely to parallel the medical adverse outcomes that are known to arise when proper medical risk assessment is not done before surgery. Unlike the universally accepted and fairly standardized processes aimed at reducing physical complications, there is no consensus on when and how PRA should be done and no guidelines exist for conducting this process. In an effort to learn more about how surgeons view this issue, the authors designed a survey addressing past experiences and current practices related to psychological screening of patients contemplating AAP.

An Institutional Review Board-approved survey form was sent to 200 randomly selected plastic and reconstructive and oral and maxillofacial surgeons distributed throughout the United States. Thirty surveys were returned completed and data were analyzed.

One in three surgeons who completed the survey admitted to having had a patient who experienced a psychological adverse outcome. In most of these cases, the patient's response was noted despite what the surgeon judged to be an acceptable surgical result. Most respondents claimed to use an intuitive sense to conduct informal PRA, and the majority stated that they seldom or never refer patients to mental health professionals. Surgeons varied in their ranking of red flags, but rated unrealistic expectations and a history of attempted suicide as the most significant. Respondents were also concerned when they believed that their patients had a discordant self-image and when patients admitted to being under psychiatric care. Eighty percent of respondents stated that they would be likely to use a tool, if one were available, to facilitate PRA.[28]

These findings are consistent with results reported in the scientific literature. In the absence of an efficient and effective method that predictably enhances the ability of the surgeon to psychologically risk stratify patients seeking AAP, most use intuitive means of conducting this assessment relying on their instinct and rarely seeking formal evaluations by mental health professionals.[12,21]

Interesting parallels are noted with bariatric surgery, a specific type of AAP that is generally limited to individuals whose obesity is a serious physical problem. The American Society of Bariatric Surgery (ASBS) has recognized the need for psychological evaluation of these patients as an important part of the preoperative assessment. In an October, 2004 report from the ad hoc behavioral health committee of the ASBS, the need for PRA in this population was acknowledged and a variety of approaches were offered from personality inventories to self-esteem and quality-of-life scales. There is a body of literature supporting the concept that, at least empirically, PRA is a critical part of the work-up for bariatric surgery.[29]

Although morbid obesity is a complex issue with significant physical implications, it is also a deformity that impacts self-image and leads affected individuals to seek change. Recognizing the differences between bariatric surgery and other AAP, it is still reasonable to draw parallels and to examine the basic principles of PRA that were developed by this behavioral health committee and are published as suggestions from the ASBS.[30]

The authors of "Suggestions for Pre-Surgical Assessment of Bariatric Surgery Candidates"[30] acknowledge the paucity of data and do not intend to have the suggestions put forth in this document viewed as best practice guidelines. However, they do make a strong case for PRA in this population, describe the elements of such a process, and discuss the value of putting the assessment into the hands of behavioral health specialists. Rather than dictate any particular testing modality, they provide a list of psychological assessment instruments that may be useful in enhancing the evaluation of surgical candidates. Several of the concepts presented in this article on the bariatric surgery subpopulation are eminently applicable to the entire population of patients who seek AAP:

- AAP may produce major benefits, but the process is likely to be stressful. As such, desirable findings during a presurgical assessment process should be a "secure identity, sound psychological resources, resiliency, effective coping strategies and willingness to access meaningful support."[30] Problematic issues should also be identified so that risk stratification can lead to appropriate intervention or to modification or deferral of the AAP.
- Categories proposed for the assessment of bariatric surgery candidates include behavioral, cognitive/emotional, developmental, current life situation, motivation, and expectations. These same areas are applicable to other AAP and are similar to the categories proposed by several authors describing PRA for orthognathic and cosmetic surgery.[20,31,32]
- For bariatric surgery candidates, psychological testing is viewed as potentially valuable to support or challenge a clinical impression and to glean information that may not have been relayed at a clinical interview. The authors of "Suggestions for Pre-Surgical Assessment of Bariatric Surgery Candidates"[30] point out that objective testing by behavioral health specialists may be a useful adjunct much in the way that laboratory testing can be an important element of the presurgical medical evaluation. Data generated by such testing might also serve to support the conclusions of behavioral health specialists in terms of risk management and professional liability. Nonetheless, they also acknowledge the absence of data supporting the use of any particular testing methods and the inappropriateness of relying on a test that may not be applicable in every situation. The use of assessment tools by psychologists is subject to the American Psychological Association's (APA) Ethics

Code. Among other recommendations made in the APA Ethics Code is the selection of assessment tools of known validity to address relevant questions.[33]

To further complicate the issue, there is a tendency among individuals undergoing psychological evaluation to distort self-reporting, either intentionally or unwittingly. In the bariatric surgery population, such distortions occur in 45% of surgical candidates.[30] Objective testing must be constructed with validity indicators designed to help determine whether or not the subject is responding honestly. Examining the role of personality inventories and similar tools in presurgical assessments for AAP, Sarwer and his associates acknowledged the limitations of such testing, citing its inability to reliably identify relevant psychopathology and predict adverse outcomes.[13,14]

SCREENING

Despite the complexities inherent in this process, surgeons and others who perform AAP seem to do a reasonable job of informal, gut feeling PRA.[21] It is unrealistic, impractical, and perhaps unnecessary to have every AAP candidate evaluated by an appropriately qualified mental health professional. Moreover, even if such an evaluation is conducted, there is no guarantee that a psychological adverse outcome will not occur. The goal is not to simply diffuse responsibility by obtaining clearance. Such an approach misses the point in the medical evaluation of the surgical patient and seems equally inappropriate for psychological assessment of patients seeking AAP. However, some screening process by the operating clinician appears to be indicated in this population. Dentists and surgeons should be able to recognize red flags, identify patients who should be evaluated by a behavioral health specialist, and, most importantly, know when to say no.

The development of a screening methodology for this purpose depends on the following:

- The process is accessible to clinicians who perform procedures and are not mental health specialists.
- The process can be conducted quickly and as a component of the work-up routinely done before elective surgery and other AAP.
- The process has the potential to assist in stratifying psychological risk as a basis for treating patients (requiring further evaluation by a mental health professional or identifying patients for whom AAP may be inappropriate).

One method that is compatible with the previously mentioned criteria is the structured interview, an approach that has been advocated in the literature on this subject despite its inherent subjectivity. Several authors have suggested areas of discussion during such an interview. There is general agreement about these areas of concern and some of the material is already routinely discussed as part of the medical/surgical interview of patients presenting for an elective AAP.[13,14,20,27,32]

The structured interview that follows is derived from the opinions and suggestions of those who have published on this subject and is proposed as one approach to data gathering relative to the emotional fitness of potential patients undergoing AAP. Scoring is based on the interviewer's impression of the answers provided by potential patients. As such, scoring is a subjective process that is affected by interviewer bias. Nonetheless, the experiences and perceptions of the interviewer are critical to the detection of patients who may benefit from a more rigorous, and possibly more objective psychological evaluation, and those for whom AAP should be denied. Despite its inherent subjectivity, the structured interview is likely to be a more sensitive screening tool than objective tests in the hands of the clinician who performs AAP.

Proposed structured interview

Ask patients when they first noticed the problem. Then ask how it has impacted the patients' life over the course of this time.

Ask patients to describe in words the level of severity of the deformity or problem.

Ask patients to explain why it is that they are seeking treatment at this time and determine whether patients have sought/had treatment for this same problem in the past. If so, get detailed information about past treatments and patients' reaction to it.

Ask patients about their relationships with other clinicians and determine if these were based in trust and understanding.

Ask patients about how comfortable they are with their physical appearance and how much time is spent mirror checking or experiencing concern about their appearance. Try to determine if dissatisfaction with appearance has affected behavior and, if so, to what extent.

Ask patients what they hope to gain from the procedure, both physically and in terms of quality of life.

Ask patients about past and present depression, suicidal ideation, psychiatric issues, therapy, and psychoactive medications, and consider whether their affect is consistent and appropriate.

Note patient behaviors/attitudes including the following:

- An inappropriate view of the clinician as a savior or the only doctor who is able to provide the desired outcome
- Attempts to manipulate or pressure the clinician
- Persistent negativity, hopelessness, and an inability to derive joy from life
- A chip on the shoulder or signs of resentment or anger
- An undue focus on physical complaints that seem unfounded
- A sense of entitlement
- An unrealistic need for perfection.

Scaling interviewer impressions for each of the previous seven items produces a score intended to assist the clinician in psychological risk stratification. Low scores are reflective of the interviewer's impression that the AAP candidate is low risk. Higher scores point to the potential benefit for a more formal evaluation by a mental health professional. The highest scores may lead a clinician to defer treatment or refer patients to a more appropriate source of care.

It should be clear that the process previously described is not a validated assessment tool. It is simply a way of collecting and organizing information in an effort to enhance a process already done informally by many clinicians who perform AAP. Moreover, its existence may stimulate thought and heighten awareness so that psychological risk assessment is considered along with well-established medical and anesthesia evaluations when contemplating elective AAP.

PRA AND THE ELECTRONIC HEALTH RECORD

Our analysis of the data is only as good as the quality of the data collected. As the electronic-health-record age continues to evolve, electronic psychological risk assessments will not only encourage more effective data collection but will provide the necessary tools to enhance the evolution of the information in many ways. Each individual clinician will have the ability to use the PRA in an electronic format that will provide a more consistent methodology for data collection, as well as the tools and reporting capabilities to assist in identifying patient profiles that may be associated with elevated risk. More concise data management can lead to refinement of the PRA process and may yield more consistent results.

The electronic health record is evolving into a system through which information may be shared among clinicians, including an interactive component that involves patients' personal health histories. This interactive functionality will provide the clinician with the ability to collect and easily share patient information with other members of the health care team. This interactivity will allow the team to use specific components, such as the PRA, in an interdisciplinary fashion to promote better overall patient management. Ultimately, a personal PRA may be used as an interactive tool to help patients understand their motivations and expectations and might even allow prospective patients to prescreen themselves at home.

SUMMARY

The need for medical and anesthetic evaluations of patients scheduled for surgery is universally recognized and has led to evidence-based guidelines. These processes are so critical that their conduct is regulated by state boards and by the Joint Commission on the Accreditation of Health care Organizations. No standard protocols or guidelines exist for the psychological screening of surgical patients, leaving this task to clinicians whose interest, training, or experience in this area may not be adequate. This lack of standards is despite compelling evidence suggesting that stratifying psychological risk before elective, appearance-altering surgery is desirable and could lead to more predictable identification of patients with an elevated risk for psychological adverse outcomes. There are significant obstacles to the development of a PRA process that parallels medical and surgical risk stratification. However, an empiric approach to psychological screening that is user friendly for dentists, surgeons, and others who perform AAP is likely to be beneficial and could be integrated into the presurgical evaluation of patients seeking esthetic surgery and other AAP.

REFERENCES

1. Kheterpal S, O'Reilly M, Englesbe MJ, et al. Preoperative and intraoperative predictors of cardiac adverse events after general, vascular and urological surgery. Anesthesiology 2009;110:58–66.
2. Smetana GW, Lawrence VA, Cornell JE. Preoperative pulmonary risk stratification for noncardiothoracic surgery: review for the American College of Physicians. Ann Intern Med 2006;144:581–95.
3. Cohn SL. Cardiac risk stratification before noncardiac surgery. Cleve Clin J Med 2006;73(Supp 1):S18–24.
4. Halaszynski TM, Juda R, Silverman DG. Optimizing postoperative outcomes with efficient preoperative assessment and management. Crit Care Med 2004;32(Supp 4):S76–86.
5. Gupta A. Preoperative screening and risk assessment in the ambulatory surgery patient. Curr Opin Anaesthesiol 2009;22:705–11.
6. Kozak EA. Preparing for surgery: this practical workup pinpoints preoperative dangers. Geriatrics 1993;48:32–45.
7. Cinello M, Nucifora G, Bertolissi M, et al. American College of Cardiology/American heart Association perioperative assessment guidleines for noncardiac surgery reduces cardiologic resource utilization preserving favourable clinical outcome. J Cardiovasc Med 2007;8:882–7.
8. Freeman WK, Gibbons RJ. Perioperative cardiovascular assessment of patients undergoing noncardiac surgery. Mayo Clin Proc. 2009;84:79–90.
9. Karnath RM. Preoperative cardiac risk assessment. Am Fam Physician 2002;66:1889–96.
10. Becker DE. Preoperative medical evaluation: part 1:general principles and cardiovascular considerations. Anesth Prog 2009;56:92–103.
11. Becker DE. Preoperative medical evaluation: part 2: pulmonary, endocrine, renal and miscellaneous considerations. Anesth Prog 2009;56:135–44.
12. Borah G, Rankin M, Wey P, et al. Psychological complications in 281 plastic surgery practices. Plast Reconstr Surg 1999;101:1241–6.
13. Sarwer DB, Pertschuk MJ, Wadden TA, et al. Psychological investigations in cosmetic surgery: a look back and a look ahead. Plast Reconstr Surg 1998;101:1136–43.
14. Crerand CE, Franklin ME, Sarwer DB. Body dysmorphic disorder and cosmetic surgery. Plast Reconstr Surg 2006;118:167e–80e.
15. Sarwer DB, Wadden TA, Pertschuk MJ, et al. Body image dissatisfaction and body dysmorphic disorder in 100 cosmetic surgery patients. Plast Reconstr Surg 1998;101:1644–9.
16. Wright MR. How to recognize and control the problem patient. J Dermatol Surg Oncol 1984;10:389–95.
17. Linn L, Goldman IB. Psychiatric observations concerning rhinoplasty. Psychol Med 1949;11:307.
18. Lipworth L, Nyren O, Ye W, et al. Excess mortality from suicide and other external causes of death among women with cosmetic breast implants. Ann Plast Surg 2007;59:569–80.
19. Gibson M, Connolly FH. The incidence of schizophrenia and severe psychological disorders in patients ten years after cosmetic rhinoplasty. Br J Plast Surg 1975;28:125–9.

20. Peterson LJ, Topazian RG. Psychological considerations in corrective maxillary and midfacial surgery. J Oral Surg 1976;34:157–64.

21. Pogrel MA, Scott P. Is it possible to identify the psychologically "bad risk" orthognathic surgery patient preoperatively? Int J Adult Orthodon Orthognath Surg 1994;9:105–10.

22. Rankin MK, Borah GL. Anxiety disorders in plastic surgery. Plast Reconstr Surg 2004;113:2199–201.

23. Honigman RJ, Phillips KA, Castle DJ. A review of psychosocial outcomes for patients seeking cosmetic surgery. Plast Reconstr Surg 2004;113:1229–37.

24. Shedler J, Westen D. Refining personality disorder diagnosis: Integrating science and practice. Am J Psychiatry 2004;161:1350–65.

25. Westen D. Divergences between clinical and research methods for assessing personality disorders: Implications for research and the evolution of axis II. Am J Psychiatry 1997;154:895–903.

26. Westen D, Shedler J. Revising and assessing axis II: Part I: developing a clinically and empirically valid assessment measure. Am J Psychiatry 1999;156:258–72.

27. Macgregor FC. Patient dissatisfaction with results of technically satisfactory surgery. Aesthetic Plast Surg 1981;5:27–32.

28. Lyne JD, Ephros HD. Psychological risk assessment for orthognathic and cosmetic surgery. J Oral Maxillofac Surg 2008;66(Suppl 1):157.

29. Gertler R, Ramsey-Stewart G. Pre-operative psychiatric assessment of patients presenting for gastric bariatric surgery. Aust N Z J Surg. 1986; 56:157–61.

30. LeMont D, Moorehead MK, Parish MS, et al, for Allied Health Sciences Section Ad Hoc Behavioral Health Committee. Suggestions for the Pre-Surgical Assessment of Bariatric Surgery Candidates. American Society for Bariatric Surgery; 2004. Available at: http://www.asbs.org/html/pdf/PsychPreSurgicalAssessment.pdf. Accessed July 17, 2010.

31. Cunningham SJ, Feinman C. Psychological assessment of patients requesting orthognathic surgery and the prevalence of body dysmorphic disorder. Br J Orthod 1998;25:293–8.

32. Thomas JR, Sclafani AP, et al. Preoperative identification of psychiatric illness in aesthetic facial surgery patients. Aesthetic Plast Surg 2001;25:64–7.

33. American Psychological Association. Ethical principals of psychologists and code of conduct. 2002 Code of Ethics. Available at: www.apa.org/ethics/code2002.html. Accessed July 17, 2010.

Psychological Risks Associated with Appearance-Altering Procedures: Issues "Facing" Cosmetic Surgery

Walter F. Ricci, MD[a,b], Steven J. Prstojevich, MD, DDS, FACS[c,d,e,f,*],
Harriet S. Langley, MD[g,h],
Matthew R. Hlavacek, MD, DDS[c,d,e,i]

KEYWORDS

- Cosmetic surgery • Psychological risk
- Shame • Mental health

Cosmetic surgery is a subspecialty that focuses on the enhancement of appearance through surgical and medical techniques. It is specifically concerned with maintaining a more youthful appearance, restoring it, or enhancing it in line with society's current aesthetic ideal. It differs from reconstructive surgery, the goal of which is to produce or restore form and function for individuals with congenital or acquired deformities and defects. Cosmetic procedures are sought by patients to alleviate symptoms of distress or dissatisfaction with their appearance.

The distress created by the perception of disfigurement or inadequacy is not always in proportion with the physical presence of disfigurement or malfunction from a clinical perspective.[1] A continuous flux occurs between the world of the subjective and the objective. People live within the selective perception that their subjective judgment accurately informs them of what is believed to be true.

Whether surgeons find the correlation between what is felt by the patient and what is observable by them to be accurate is a key issue in deciding whether there is an indication for treatment and in establishing the therapeutic alliance between doctor and patient and the patient's satisfaction, or lack of it, with the outcome of the surgery.

[a] Department of Psychiatry, University of Missouri-Kansas City, School of Medicine, Kansas City, MO, USA
[b] Greater Kansas City Psychoanalytic Institute, Kansas City, MO, USA
[c] Department of Oral and Maxillofacial Surgery, University of Missouri-Kansas City, School of Medicine, 2411 Holmes Street, Kansas City, MO 64108-2784, USA
[d] Department of Oral and Maxillofacial Surgery, University of Missouri-Kansas City, School of Dentistry, 650 East 25th Street, Kansas City, MO 64108-2784, USA
[e] Facial and Cosmetic Surgery, St Luke's Hospital, 4401 Wornall, Kansas City, MO 64111, USA
[f] Oral and Maxillofacial Surgery, University of Missouri-Kansas City, St Luke's Hospital, 4401 Wornall, Kansas City, MO 64111, USA
[g] Department of Medicine, University of Missouri-Kansas City School of Medicine, Kansas City, MO, USA
[h] Menorah Medical Center, 5721 West 119th Street, Overland Park, KS 66209-3722, USA
[i] Department of Surgery, University of Missouri-Kansas City, School of Medicine, Kansas City, MO, USA
* Corresponding author. Department of Oral and Maxillofacial Surgery, University of Missouri-Kansas City, School of Medicine, 2411 Holmes Street, Kansas City, MO 64108-2784.
E-mail address: face@sbcglobal.net

Oral Maxillofacial Surg Clin N Am 22 (2010) 439–444
doi:10.1016/j.coms.2010.07.010
1042-3699/10/$ — see front matter © 2010 Elsevier Inc. All rights reserved.

PSYCHOLOGICAL ASPECTS OF COSMETIC SURGERY PATIENTS

All individuals have a repertoire of coping devices or defenses that allows them to maintain equilibrium between what drives them internally and the world around them. This repertoire creates the characteristics of their personality, which, in turn, dictates their lifestyles.

All individuals as part of humankind live connected to some standard of beauty and perfection. Whether or not they are aware of it, there is a system and powerful structure in their minds, which is quickly activated if there is a gap in or deviation from their pre-established standards and values. The distance between that standard and the one of their actual performance or appearance, objectively or subjectively appraised, comes to be experienced as a state of pride or shame. At times, adherence to this feeling could be so tenacious that it acquires the quasi-delusional intensity of an unshakeable, erroneous, or pathologic belief that guides the individual's thoughts and actions.

People adopt different strategies to defend against the experience of shame, which may alter their behavior. Nathanson[2] describes 4 different strategies to deal with the affect of shame when it becomes unbearable, illustrated in **Fig. 1** and described in the following text:

1. At the withdrawal pole of the compass, people tend to withdraw and hide. Nathanson says, "the most benign behaviors of the withdrawal pole of the compass involves such gestures as putting hands to lips as if to prevent or retract whatever has been said." He adds, "At the pathologic end are all the ways we hide from those who represent harm," such as impotence, frigidity, and reclusive behavior.

2. The attack-self pole is diminishing oneself as the price of maintaining connection with another person. Nathanson provides, "how could you want to be with someone as horrible as me?" Other examples are relationships of chronic abuse and masochism.

3. In the avoidance pole, there are moments when one simply cannot tolerate the recognition of shame and one does anything to prevent that experience by calling attention to whatever brings one pride, such as owning exotic cars, trophies, and jewelry, undergoing cosmetic surgery, or achieving physical fitness beyond the norm. One also includes ways to block the physiologic experience of shame with drugs, alcohol, hedonism, or other self-destructive behaviors.

4. The attack other pole of the compass includes all the systems of behavior we use to reduce, humiliate, abuse, or torture those with whom we conflictively interact. As the author states, "I increase my self esteem by reducing someone else".

Thus, any experience that engages the evaluation of the physical or psychological self according to a positive or negative value is subjectively felt as deadening or enlivening by the experiencing person. Like an inexorable law, whatever does not increase one's pride increases one's shame or embarrassment, requiring the development of coping tactics or maneuvers to deal with it.

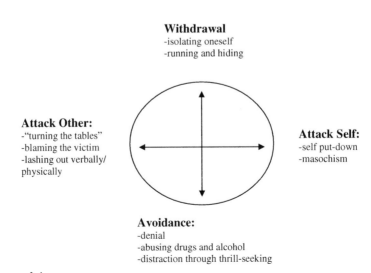

Fig. 1. The compass of shame.

SENSE OF IDENTITY

Physiognomy is a word from the Greek "physis" meaning "nature" and "gnomon" meaning "judge." It is generally defined as the appraisal of people's character from their outer appearance, especially their faces. This relationship between the outer appearance and the inner character and the perceived aesthetic value given by society's customs and fashions exert a powerful influence on the life and destiny of the individual.[3]

Erickson[4] described identity as being based on 2 basic observations: (1) the immediate perception of one's self-sameness and continuity in time; and, (2) the experience that others recognize one's sameness and continuity, thus confirming and validating one's identity.

This sense of continuity could be disrupted by disfiguring accidents, events, or conditions. Conversely, features that are unwanted, such as wrinkles, sagging tissue, or fat deposits, benefit from changes that enhance our subjectively perceived appearance. Thus, restoration or transformation become part of the key goals of the individual and lead to the need to seek help from the surgeon, the psychologist, or both.

SPECTRUM OF NARCISSISM

The presence of narcissism is a normal component of any personality type. It is part of one's self-survival/preservation and serves as a regulator of healthy self-esteem, ambitions, and ideals. First described by Ellis in 1858, narcissistic is a term that Freud used in 1910 in a footnote to the "Three essays on the theory of sexuality." Although this term is used pejoratively today as a synonym for self-centeredness, initially it was considered in psychoanalysis to be part of the normal developmental stage in children. Secondary narcissism indicates an unusual degree of attention or preoccupation or energy directed exclusively toward oneself.

The condition becomes pathologic when it impairs social interpersonal functioning and excludes the recognition and importance of others. Thus, the narcissistic individual imbued with a sense of specialness, self-importance, omnipotence, and uniqueness has little interest or energy in recognizing the existence of other human beings. Consequently, the other person's initiatives, motivations, or preferences are of little value. Narcissistic individuals are fueled by the desire for perfection and power. The differences between their own expectations and those of other people typically evoke a response by the narcissist with unacknowledged shame,[5] defended vigorously by anger, indifference, contempt, and devaluation of others and their views. Narcissists need validation of their special status and require this with the intensity of addicts: the presence of a "public or audience." This object or person must reflect back to them the self-perceived greatness, power, and superior status to which they are rightfully entitled in their own eyes. These patients, when visiting the cosmetic surgeon's office, could create serious tensions and conflicts in the relationship while seeking the help of the surgeon to enhance and achieve that standard of perfection that is being sought.

The demanding, narcissistic patient may operate from the position that denies completely the possibility of conceiving the subjectivity and opinions of the surgeon. In this way, the patient may not be able to tolerate any expected lack of control over the professional's behavior or the desired outcome. Narcissistic rage is the name given by Heinz Kohut[6] to the sudden fury connected with the recognition that the other, in this case, the surgeon or surgeon's staff, is not acting as an extension of the narcissist's self. The narcissist expects total control, usually the kind of control one expects to have over one's own extremities. This predisposed nature unleashes fury destined to obliterate the other, in this case, the surgeon, for not giving the narcissist the outcome required. The narcissistically challenged patient's expectation is highly vulnerable to disappointment and its consequences.

THE GESTALT OF THE PATIENT, SURGEON, ANCILLARY STAFF, AND HEALTH CARE SURROUNDINGS

The assessment of the totality of the situation should include the personality of the surgeon, the professional staff involved with patient care, and the overall ambiance of the office. Any of these components have the potential to interact and create an emotional explosion. Ideally, all individuals need to be cognizant of their contribution to the overall professional relationship. If the surgeon's omnipotence overrules his or her limitations or obscures good judgment about the feasibility of the procedure, a dangerous situation is created. Humility and recognition of the surgeon's own therapeutic skill is paramount. What a surgeon may lack in empathy is hopefully offset by the care and compassion of the staff. In addition, the warmth of the actual physical setting helps provide a nurturing environment.

Like the patient seeking the procedure to enhance self-esteem, surgeons should be aware that as human beings and professionals, they are also seeking validation of their work and reward, and only through self-reflection can the surgeon assess the different factors involved in the treatment of the patient. These factors include

1. the patient's perception of the problem
2. the patient's personality
3. the context of and events occurring in the patient's life at the time of any health care encounters
4. the surgeon's proven skills in the procedure
5. the surgeon's personality
6. the context of and events, both professional and personal, occurring in the surgeon's life at the time of any patient interaction
7. the direct, humble, and realistic promise of what might be safely delivered.

THE RELATIONSHIP BETWEEN SURGEON AND PATIENT

The relationship between surgeon and patient should be seen from the perspective of both recognizing each other as subjects. When one is being related to as a subject, it is a feeling of being understood or "felt" by the other. There may be gaps or ruptures in this feeling, but there should always be a genuine attempt to repair that rupture and reestablish the mutuality of human validation. Many studies establish that doctors who are being perceived as authoritarian, contemptuous, or dismissive in their encounters with their patients are sued more often than those who are empathic in their care and approach.[8]

Perceiving each other as subjects is an absolute condition for collaboration and the development of a symbiotic relationship. The asymmetry in the relationship exists only in the technical and professional realm. The surgeon possesses the skill, the knowledge, and hopefully, the empathy needed by the patient. The patient offers the opportunity for physicians to use their experience and skills, and in so doing, the clinician gains esteem and other rewards. The recognition of the mutuality of the human condition is the most basic element of the relationship. Under no circumstances can this human condition be skewed or diminished without objectification being the outcome, leading to shame and its consequences.

EXPECTATIONS OF OUTCOME

The outcome of and degree of satisfaction with appearance-altering procedures is related to several factors. The degree of improvement or enhancement of self-esteem in the patient can depend on the type of surgery involved and the changes from previous images. Surgeries such as rhinoplasty are more difficult to assimilate or accommodate by some patients, with the changes in body image, because the outcome can be a new, previously unimagined look.[9] Other procedures more reconstructive in nature may be easier to assimilate. The patient's or partner's expectations play a very important role in the acceptance of the outcome. Was the surgery really initiated by the patient from within or was it a product of external motivation?

The following cases help to illustrate the complexity of the evaluation process required for patients seeking elective surgical procedures.

Clinical Vignette 1

C is a 41-year-old businessman who was referred to the psychiatrist's office by his internist. He was diagnosed with a social phobia and believed that his career was derailed because of his shyness. Further into the evaluation, he shared the fact that he had gynecomastia, which he painfully admitted prevented him from participating in business social activities and corporation team building events in which he had to remove his shirt. He was on serotonin inhibitors for the treatment of what was thought to be social phobia.

After exploring difficult issues through psychoanalysis, he was referred for cosmetic surgery consultation. The surgeon recommended liposuction of his chest, which C underwent. Postoperatively, he felt relieved and proud of the results achieved by the surgery. He felt his life had a new beginning, and he sensed that this would allow him to more readily reach his personal and professional goals.

Clinical Vignette 2

M is a 34-year-old woman who was referred to a psychiatrist for evaluation. The referral was made by a cosmetic surgeon from whom she was requesting breast augmentation surgery. M was a very attractive and shapely woman. During the interview, she revealed a history of child abuse and multiple failed relationships. She showed signs of depression and feelings of hopelessness and a lack of zest for living. Later in the interview, she stated that she was satisfied with her figure and with the size of her breasts. It was revealed that her boyfriend was pressing her, with the threat of abandonment, to undergo this surgery. She was a former exotic dancer currently in college, which was partially paid for by her boyfriend. He envisioned her going back to her old job.

Psychotherapy along with psychotropic drugs was recommended and surgery was postponed until she was able to make a more independent decision.

The correction of some perceived deficiency or defect that has an important value as a provider of self-esteem may be an important and primary goal sought by the patient. In appropriately selected cases, the surgical outcome may have a significant positive impact on the patient's life. However, in patients with difficulties regulating self-esteem, having a positive outcome from surgical changes cannot be taken for granted. Surgery may lead to disappointments, depression, new surgical attempts, or legal action.

PSYCHIATRIC ISSUES THAT REQUIRE SPECIAL CONSIDERATION FOR THE SURGICAL PATIENT

Among the main issues involved in the satisfactory outcome of surgery are the mental health factors of patients seeking cosmetic surgery. Up to 47.7% of patients who consult for cosmetic procedures meet criteria for having a mental disorder.[10] These include body dysmorphic disorder (BDD),[7] which occurs in 5% to 15% of patients; narcissistic personality disorder (NPD), in 25%, and histrionic personality disorders, in 9.7%.[11] Given the prevalence of these disorders, the importance of having a clear evaluation of the patient seeking surgery becomes apparent.

BDD (*Diagnostic and Statistical Manual of Mental Disorders, Fourth Edition* [DSM-IV])[12] is a type of somatoform disorder.

This condition is described as one in which patients have an imagined defect in appearance. If there is even a slight physical defect, the patients' concern about it is excessively exaggerated. The preoccupation causes significant distress or impairment in the patient's social, occupational, or other important areas of functioning.

The preoccupation is not better accounted for by another mental disorder, such as dissatisfaction with body shape and size as in anorexia nervosa. According to David Veale,[13] screening for this condition involves asking the following questions:

1. Do you currently think a lot about your appearance?
2. What features are you happy with? Do you feel your features are unattractive?
3. How abnormal or noticeable do you think your features are?
4. How much time do you spend on thinking about this feature or checking on it?
5. Does this feature affect your social life in that you avoid encounters?
6. Does your feature interfere with your ability to work or study or relate to others?

Many of the dynamic features of NPD have been outlined above and in related articles in this journal. According to DSM IV, individuals with NPD display "a pervasive pattern of grandiosity (in fantasy or behavior), a need for admiration, or lack of empathy beginning in early adulthood and present in a variety of contexts."[12] Key traits are

1. grandiose sense of self-importance
2. preoccupation with unlimited power, success, brilliance, beauty, and so forth
3. sense of specialness
4. requiring continuous admiring responses
5. sense of entitlement
6. interpersonal exploitative behavior
7. lack of empathy
8. envy of others or vice versa
9. arrogance or haughty behavior.

Another personality disorder of interest to clinicians performing appearance-altering procedures is the histrionic type. The DSM IV describes this as "a pervasive pattern of excessive emotionally and attention-seeking behavior beginning by early adulthood and present in a variety of contexts."[12] Findings include

1. unhappiness in situations in which they are not the center of attention
2. inappropriate sexually seductive provocative behavior
3. rapidly shifting and shallow expressions of emotion
4. use of physical appearance to draw attention to self
5. style of speech excessively impressionistic and lacking in detail
6. dramatization, theatricality, excessive display of emotions
7. suggestibility
8. professing more intimacy in relations than is actually there.

There are other patients with certain conditions that should be carefully screened, because their mental and emotional status may impair their judgment. Such conditions include psychosis, certain borderline disorders with liability of mood, severe eating disorders, chronic depression, and surgery addictions, a subclass of Munchausen syndrome. It is extremely important to try to quantify the patient's present stability, degree of resilience, and ability to cope with complications and less than desirable outcomes. Consequently, a carefully recorded medical and social history and a skillful psychological evaluation should be a basic requirement before performing any appearance-altering surgical procedures.

Special attention should be given to patients who have had multiple previous surgical treatments. Patients' issues with the previous procedures and surgeons should be meticulously appraised and evaluated. Is the patient's understanding based on sound psychological-mindedness? Are the patients capable of insight and comprehension of the intricacies of the surgeries to which they are consenting?

Surgeon should be advised not to rely only on the opinion of those who make the psychological assessment; rather, they should also have formed their own overall impression (gestalt) obtained during the consultation. Is the patient excessively dependent, anxious, demanding, or depressed? Does the patient have adequate coping defense mechanisms? Does the patient have realistic expectations?

Is the patient on the verge of psychological fragmentation or on the verge of rage or using seductive behavior? Whatever the factors, there should be a careful match between the difficulties of the procedure and the psychological burden of the surgery.

SUMMARY

There is a dynamic and fluid relationship between cosmetic surgery and psychology that requires careful and constant attention from the surgeon. Surgeons all desire a "short and sweet" checklist evaluation that tells them if it is safe for the patient to undergo an elective surgical procedure. Obviously, this is wishful thinking. It is asking too much for surgeons to be able to quantify the overall psychological risk. Rather, they should objectively screen, review, and evaluate as many of the variables as possible. These include but are not limited to the surgical issue, the personality of the patient, the patient's family and/or relationships, and the overall context of the situation. Surgeons should also reflect on both their technical expertise and limitations and the patient's personal resiliency.

Once everything is considered, surgeons can better determine if they should proceed with treatment or refer the patient to a mental health care provider.

REFERENCES

1. Ong J, Clarke A, White P, et al. Does severity predict distress? The relationship between subjective and objective measures of appearance and psychological adjustment, during treatment for facial lipoatrophy. Body Image 2007;4:239–48.
2. Nathanson D, W.W Norton & Company New York London. Shame and pride 1992;22(4):305–14.
3. Amodeo CA. The central role of the nose in the face and the psyche: review of the nose and the psyche. Aesthetic Plast Surg 2007;31:406–10.
4. Erickson EH. The problem of ego identity. J Am Psychoanal Assoc 1956;4:56–121.
5. Lewis HB. Shame and Guilt in Neurosis. New York: International Universities Press; 1971.
6. Kohut H. In: Ornetein P, editor. Thoughts on Narcissism and Narcissistic rage in: the search for the self. New York: International Universities Press; 1992. p. 615–62.
7. Ricci W, Broucek F. Neutrality, abstinence, and anonymity revisited. Seventeenth Annual Conference of the psychology of the Self. Chicago, October 21, 1994.
8. Gladwell M. Blink: the power of thinking without thinking. New York: Little, Brown, & Company; 2006. p. 41–3.
9. Ambro BT, Wright RJ. Psychological considerations in revision rhinoplasty. Facial Plast Surg 2008;24(3):288–92.
10. Ishigooka J, Iwao M, Suzuki M, et al. Demographic features of patients seeking cosmetic surgery. Psychiatry Clin Neurosci 1998;52:283–7.
11. Mallick F, Howard J, Koo J. Understanding the psychology of the cosmetic patients. Dermatologic Ther 2008;21:47–53.
12. Diagnostic Criteria from DSM-IV-TR. Arlington (VA): American Psychiatric Association; 2000.
13. Veale D. Psychological aspects of a cosmetic procedure. J Psychiatr Med 2006;5(3):93–4.

Body Dysmorphic Disorder in Patients Who Seek Appearance-Enhancing Medical Treatments

David B. Sarwer, PhD[a,b,*], Canice E. Crerand, PhD[c],
Leanne Magee, PhD[c]

KEYWORDS

- Body dysmorphic disorder • Maxillofacial surgery
- Body image dissatisfaction • Psychiatric disorders

In the past several years, there has been a greater appreciation of the interaction between medical illness and psychosocial factors. This relationship is of particular interest to medical professionals, such as plastic surgeons, dermatologists, and oral and maxillofacial surgeons, who perform procedures that affect physical appearance. For the patients of these providers, psychosocial rather than functional concerns are often the primary motivation for treatment. Similarly, the impact of these treatments may be greater in the psychosocial rather than physical realm.

Body image dissatisfaction seems to be common among patients who seek appearance-enhancing medical treatments. However, some individuals present with extreme levels of body image dissatisfaction suggestive of the psychiatric diagnosis of body dysmorphic disorder (BDD). This article provides an overview of BDD for the non–mental health professional. The authors review the diagnostic criteria, causes, and clinical and demographic characteristics of the disorder. The prevalence of BDD in medical populations is highlighted as is the evidence suggesting that the vast majority of persons with BDD who receive appearance-enhancing medical treatments report dissatisfaction with their outcomes and no improvement in BDD symptoms. The article concludes with a discussion of issues related to patient and provider safety.

PSYCHIATRIC DISORDERS AMONG PERSONS SEEKING APPEARANCE-ENHANCING MEDICAL TREATMENTS

Since the late 1950s, there has been an interest in the psychological characteristics of persons who undergo cosmetic surgery and other appearance-enhancing medical treatments. As we have detailed elsewhere,[1–8] although this long legacy of research has increased the understanding of some of the psychiatric conditions

[a] Division of Plastic Surgery, Department of Surgery, The Edwin and Fannie Gray Hall Center for Human Appearance, The University of Pennsylvania School of Medicine, 10 Penn Tower, 3400 Spruce Street, Philadelphia, PA 19104, USA
[b] Department of Psychiatry, Center for Weight and Eating Disorders, The University of Pennsylvania School of Medicine, 10 Penn Tower, 3400 Spruce Street, Philadelphia, PA 19104, USA
[c] Division of Plastic and Reconstructive Surgery, Department of Psychology, The Edwin and Fannie Gray Hall Center for Human Appearance, The Children's Hospital of Philadelphia, Wood Ambulatory Care Building, First Floor, 34th and Civic Center Boulevard, Philadelphia, PA 19104, USA
* Corresponding author.
E-mail address: dsarwer@mail.med.upenn.edu

Oral Maxillofacial Surg Clin N Am 22 (2010) 445–453
doi:10.1016/j.coms.2010.07.002
1042-3699/10/$ — see front matter © 2010 Published by Elsevier Inc.

relevant to these patient populations, methodological limitations have limited the ability to draw firm conclusions from this body of work. Thus, with few exceptions, the authors have not yet reached the point whereby they can state, with a good degree of confidence, that certain psychological characteristics or psychiatric diagnoses are associated with poor postoperative outcomes.

Within the past 2 decades, research on the psychological functioning of individuals who seek appearance-enhancing treatments has shifted its focus to understanding the relationship between body image and these procedures. Body image is a psychological construct defined as perceptions, thoughts, feelings, and behaviors about the body and bodily experiences.[4,8,9] Body image dissatisfaction predicts interest in cosmetic surgery.[10–12] Cosmetic surgery patients typically experience heightened body image dissatisfaction before surgery,[9,13–16] and studies have documented improvements in body image postoperatively.[17–25] The impact of cosmetic surgery on other areas of psychological functioning, such as quality of life and self-esteem, is less well understood.

Although some degree of body image dissatisfaction is typical among cosmetic surgery patients, some patients present for treatment with an excessive degree of dissatisfaction with their appearance. Significant body image dissatisfaction is a symptom of several psychiatric disorders, most notably eating disorders such as anorexia nervosa. It is also one of the defining characteristics of body dysmorphic disorder (BDD).

DIAGNOSTIC CRITERIA FOR BDD

BDD is characterized by an excessive preoccupation with an imagined or slight defect in appearance, which results in clinically significant distress and impairment in functioning.[26] The diagnosis of this condition requires the presence of perceptual inaccuracy regarding one's appearance (usually a core cognitive distortion of being misshapen, deformed, ugly, or unattractive) and extreme and negative value judgments about the appearance feature, which lead to obsessive preoccupation and interference in daily functioning. Patients with BDD report that they worry about their perceived appearance flaws several hours a day, and more than half hold on to their distorted beliefs with delusional intensity.[27]

BDD seems to be a common but underdiagnosed disorder in psychiatric settings,[28–30] in cosmetic surgery and dermatology practices,[9,31–35] as well as in orthodontic and oral and maxillofacial surgery settings.[36–40] Although some cases of BDD are easy to identify, the diagnosis can be challenging to make among persons who present for appearance-enhancing medical treatments.[1,2,5,31] Some individuals who pursue these treatments are interested in correcting slight defects in appearance or improving otherwise normal features. There can be a great deal of subjectivity on the part of both the patient and the treatment provider regarding normality of an individual's appearance or whether a particular feature can be medically corrected. Furthermore, the degree of distress associated with the feature can fall on a wide continuum. Individuals who have dropped out of school because of appearance concerns likely meet the criteria for BDD. However, persons who report some situation-specific self-consciousness because of their appearance, but are functioning appropriately in other areas of life, likely do not have BDD. Nevertheless, the authors believe that the degree of distress and functional impairment may be the most accurate indicators of BDD.[1,3,8,41]

ETIOLOGIC FACTORS OF BDD

BDD is believed to develop as a result of multiple factors.[42] Cognitive and neurobiological abnormalities have been implicated in the cause and maintenance of BDD symptoms. Individuals with BDD tend to overfocus on minor defects and ignore the global aspects of appearance.[43,44] Imaging studies have identified deficits in verbal and nonverbal memory skills and organizational encoding abilities, as well as abnormalities in the frontostriatal system and the parietal region of the brain, among individuals with BDD.[43,45–47] In addition, persons with BDD seem to respond preferentially to medications that alter the levels of dopamine and serotonin,[45] suggesting that these neurotransmitters may be involved in the disorder. Other research focusing on genetic factors has found that 20% of persons with BDD have at least 1 first-degree family member with the disorder.[48] BDD also seems to be common in families of individuals with obsessive-compulsive disorder (OCD), a finding that suggests the potential for a shared genetic link for these disorders.[49]

The development of BDD can also be understood from a psychosocial perspective. Although initial descriptions from decades ago suggested that BDD develops from unconscious displacement of sexual or emotional conflict or feelings of inferiority, guilt, or poor self-image onto a body part, such theories have garnered no empiric support.[9] Rather, more contemporary research suggests that BDD arises from an interaction of cognitive, emotional, and behavioral factors.[50,51] This approach has some empiric support, as has been reviewed in detail elsewhere.[1,2]

CLINICAL AND DEMOGRAPHIC FEATURES OF BDD

Persons with BDD typically report preoccupation with their skin, hair, and nose[48,52]; other frequently reported areas of concern include teeth, stomach, and weight.[53] However, any body part can become a source of preoccupation, and persons with BDD typically develop concerns with multiple body parts.[48] Individuals with BDD may report distinct concerns (eg, concerns about 1 or 2 teeth); others present with vague complaints (eg, concerns that a body part is ugly).[54] Preoccupations with one body part may disappear and shift to another feature over time.[54]

Individuals with BDD typically experience obsessive thoughts about their appearance that are difficult to control, particularly in situations in which the person feels self-conscious or expects to be scrutinized.[55,56] In severe cases, it can be difficult for persons with BDD to think about anything other than their appearance concerns. Patients also frequently engage in compulsive, ritualized behaviors that consume inordinate amounts of time and significantly interfere with social and occupational functioning. Most of these behaviors are performed in an effort to inspect, improve, or camouflage the area of preoccupation.[29] People with BDD typically engage in these behaviors because they mistakenly believe that their actions reduce their appearance-related distress. Unfortunately, these behaviors often increase their degree of preoccupation and, ultimately, distress. In some instances, persons with BDD have become so distressed about their defects that they have attempted to perform do-it-yourself cosmetic procedures.[57] Suicidal ideation and suicide attempts are also common among persons with BDD.[29,58-60] Some may become hostile and physically violent, directing this anger at others, including treating physicians.[48,61-64]

The typical age of onset of BDD is 16 years.[65,66] However, most individuals with BDD do not seek psychiatric treatment until their early 30s.[65,66] This is often a function of misdiagnosis, as BDD is frequently misdiagnosed. BDD seems to occur with similar frequency among women and men,[26,66] although some studies have reported higher rates among women,[48] and others, a higher rate among men.[55,67] BDD typically has a continuous rather than an episodic course.[48]

PSYCHIATRIC COMORBIDITY WITH BDD

BDD typically occurs with several comorbid psychiatric conditions. The most common is major depression, with rates ranging from 36% to 90%.[2] Anxiety disorders are also common, with 30% to 40% of patients reporting social phobia and OCD. BDD may also co-occur with obsessive-compulsive spectrum disorders, including tricho-tillomania (repetitive hair pulling), skin picking, pathologic gambling, tic disorders, and compulsive shopping.[1,2]

Individuals with BDD often suffer from substance abuse problems. Between 25% and 49% of persons with BDD have lifetime histories of substance use disorders, and 13% to 17% meet current diagnostic criteria.[68,69] Eating disorders, such as anorexia and bulimia, are also common, with lifetime rates of 7% to 14% and current rates of 4% reported among individuals with BDD.[68] Personality disorders are also quite common among persons with BDD.[66,70-72]

PREVALENCE OF BDD

In community samples, the prevalence of BDD has ranged from 0.7% to 3%.[49,73-75] Between 2% and 5% of high school and college students seem to meet diagnostic criteria.[10,76-80] However, studies of medical populations suggest much higher rates of BDD. Among patients requesting reconstructive surgical procedures, 7% to 16% reported appearance preoccupation and distress consistent with BDD.[35,81] A rate of 7.5% has been reported in patients presenting for orthodontic treatment.[37] A recent study of 160 patients presenting for maxillofacial procedures found that 10% of the patients met the criteria for BDD.[36] Case reports have also described patients with BDD in dental practices,[82,83] maxillofacial surgery clinics,[38,39] and orthognathic surgery populations.[40]

Several studies throughout the world have investigated the rate of BDD among cosmetic surgery and dermatology patients. Studies have suggested that between 3% and 17% of persons who present for cosmetic surgery have BDD.[9,67,84-91] Variability in the rates is likely a function of studies, which have focused on all cosmetic patients (vs specific procedures) and have used different assessment methods to determine the diagnosis. Studies of dermatology populations suggest similar rates, typically from 8.5% to 15%.[32,33,36,92]

TREATMENT OF BDD

As individuals with BDD believe that their appearance defects are responsible for their distress, many seek appearance-enhancing medical treatments. It seems that these treatments rarely result in an improvement in symptoms and may contribute to a worsening of the disorder. Among individuals with BDD, 71% have sought cosmetic treatments and 64% have received them.[93] Dermatologic and surgical procedures were among the most frequently sought and received procedures.[52,65,93,94] Unfortunately, most patients who receive these treatments experience poor outcomes.[52,66,93,95] Studies suggest that greater than 90% of cosmetic treatments typically produce no change, or even worse, an exacerbation of BDD symptoms.[66,93]

Although persons with BDD frequently seek these treatments, physicians seem to have some awareness of the disorder. In a survey of aesthetic surgeons completed almost 10 years ago, 84% indicated that they had not operated on a patient they suspected of having BDD.[68] Most professionals surveyed reported that they had the unfortunate experience of treating a patient who was discovered to have BDD after treatment.[68] As detailed later in the discussion, these patients can create several challenges for the surgeon and staff.[96] At a minimum, they may become a significant management issue. Others may be more likely to threaten or execute lawsuits against their physicians. There are documented cases of physicians who have been murdered by patients who had symptoms consistent with BDD.[97]

For these reasons, coupled with the evidence that cosmetic treatments rarely improve BDD symptoms, there is growing consensus that BDD should be considered a contraindication for cosmetic treatments.[31,52,66,93,95,98–100] Psychiatric and psychotherapeutic treatments seem to be far more effective in treating BDD. Both open-label and randomized controlled trials have demonstrated the efficacy of selective serotonin reuptake inhibitor (SSRI) medications in the treatment of BDD.[54,101–109] Despite these promising findings, BDD remains a challenging disorder to treat. Patients treated with SSRIs may exhibit only partial responses to treatment, and many require long trials and high dosages of multiple SSRIs to experience symptom relief. Other patients benefit from augmentation with antipsychotic medications if they have delusional symptoms. Cognitive behavioral therapy (CBT), a type of psychotherapy that involves the identifying and changing problematic appearance-related thoughts and behaviors, has been found to be an efficacious treatment for BDD in several studies.[56,60,110–112] According to a meta-analysis of psychological and pharmacologic treatments for BDD, CBT seems to yield even greater symptom improvements in comparison to pharmacotherapy.[113]

MANAGEMENT OF BDD IN ORAL AND MAXILLOFACIAL SURGERY PRACTICE

Given the popularity of appearance-enhancing medical treatments and the frequency with which persons with BDD pursue them, oral and maxillofacial surgeons are likely to encounter patients who present with symptoms of BDD. Because of the aforementioned safety concerns associated with treating persons with BDD, it is important that all patients be assessed for BDD before treatment. Pretreatment screening can help identify symptoms, safeguard providers against patients who could become litigious or violent, and direct patients to appropriate treatments.

As detailed elsewhere,[1–5,7,31,35,96] a general psychological screening, consisting of an assessment of patient motivations and expectations for the procedure, appearance concerns and BDD symptoms, psychiatric status and history, and observations of the patient's behavior at the office, can identify persons for whom treatment may be inappropriate.[96,114,115] Asking new patients about their motivations and expectations regarding surgery may uncover potential indicators of BDD. Patients who report that they expect surgery to transform their lives or who express other unrealistic beliefs (eg, surgery will save a failing marriage) may be suffering from BDD.[96,97]

Oral and maxillofacial surgeons or designated staff members should specifically inquire about appearance concerns and BDD symptoms, including the degree of distress that the patients have about their appearance and how this interferes with their daily functioning and interpersonal relationships. Patients should be able to discuss specific oral appearance concerns that are readily observable. Patients with a relatively normal appearance who report significant distress or who indicate that their preoccupation with appearance interferes with daily functioning may be suffering from BDD. Other indicators of BDD include excessive camouflaging (eg, a patient hiding her mouth behind her hand when she speaks), avoidance of social activities, or an inability to maintain relationships or employment because of appearance concerns.

A patient's medical history may also offer clues about BDD. Patients who indicate that they have undergone prior or repeated dental or oral surgical treatments or who report dissatisfaction with previous procedures should be carefully screened. A psychiatric treatment history, including direct questions about the patient's history of psychopharmacologic and psychotherapeutic treatments as well as psychiatric hospitalizations, should be obtained. Because BDD typically co-occurs with other psychiatric disorders, particularly depression, patients who present with current symptoms or a history of psychiatric disorders should be assessed for BDD. Patients who present with a history of psychopathology but are not currently engaged in any type of treatment should undergo a preoperative psychiatric consultation. For patients who are engaged in psychiatric or psychological treatment, the oral and maxillofacial surgeon or staff should contact the patient's mental health care provider to verify that surgery is appropriate at this time. Assessing for psychiatric disorders is additionally important given that some patients who have been dissatisfied with their postoperative results have used their psychiatric history as part of their legal action against their surgeon, claiming that their psychiatric condition prevented them from fully understanding the procedure and potential outcomes.[96]

A patient's behavior in the office may also suggest the presence of BDD or other psychopathology.[96] Because patients are frequently on their best behavior when meeting with the physicians, office staff and nurses may observe different aspects of patients' behavior, which may offer clues about potential problems. Staff may notice unusual requests for appointment times, excessive phone calls, or other deviations from standard procedures, which could be indicative of BDD. Nurses may notice inconsistencies in the patient's reports or other atypical behaviors, such as excessive seeking of reassurance, which may be suggestive of psychopathology. A second consultation is appropriate for patients who raise concerns among the office staff. After the second consultation with the surgeon, if concerns continue to exist, a mental health evaluation is recommended.

SUMMARY

Over the past 2 decades, a great deal has been learned about the importance of psychosocial factors in medical treatment. In the realm of medical treatments that affect physical appearance, such as oral and maxillofacial surgery, much of this focus has been on body image. Most patients who seek appearance-enhancing medical treatments report some degree of body image dissatisfaction, which is believed to motivate the pursuit of these treatments. However, those with extreme body image dissatisfaction may be suffering from BDD. This condition is seen far more commonly among persons interested in cosmetic procedures than in the general population. Unfortunately, appearance-enhancing treatments seem to have little effect on the symptoms of BDD. Anecdotal reports suggest that patients with BDD may become litigious, threaten, or actually commit acts of violence directed at the treating physician. For these reasons, BDD is considered by many to be a contraindication to cosmetic procedures. Oral and maxillofacial surgeons and other clinicians who offer appearance-enhancing treatments should routinely screen for BDD symptoms and refer patients suspected of suffering from the disorder for additional mental health evaluation before treatment.

REFERENCES

1. Crerand CE, Franklin ME, Sarwer DB. Body dysmorphic disorder and cosmetic surgery. Plast Reconstr Surg 2006;118:167e–80e.
2. Sarwer DB, Crerand CE. Body dysmorphic disorder and appearance-enhancing medical treatments. Body Image 2008;5:50–8.
3. Crerand CE, Cash TF, Whitaker LA. Cosmetic surgery of the face. In: Sarwer DB, Pruzinsky T, Cash TF, et al, editors. Psychological aspects of reconstructive and cosmetic plastic surgery: clinical, empirical and ethical perspectives. Philadelphia: Lippincott Williams & Wilkins; 2006. p. 233–49.
4. Sarwer DB, Crerand CE. Body image and cosmetic medical treatments. Body Image 2004;1:99–111.
5. Sarwer DB, Crerand CE, Gibbons LM. Body dysmorphic disorder. In: Nahai F, editor. The art of aesthetic surgery. St Louis (MO): Quality Medical Publishing; 2006. p. 33–57.
6. Sarwer DB, Didie ER, Gibbons LM. Cosmetic surgery of the body. In: Sarwer DB, Pruzinsky T, Cash TF, et al, editors. Psychological aspects of reconstructive and cosmetic plastic surgery: clinical, empirical and ethical perspectives. Philadelphia: Lippincott Williams & Wilkins; 2006. p. 251–66.
7. Sarwer DB, Magee L, Crerand CE. Cosmetic surgery and cosmetic medical treatments. In: Thompson KA, editor. Handbook of eating disorders and obesity. Hoboken (NJ): John Wiley & Sons, Inc; 2004. p. 718–37.
8. Sarwer DB, Wadden TA, Pertschuk MJ, et al. The psychology of cosmetic surgery: a review and reconceptualization. Clin Psychol Rev 1998;18:1–22.
9. Sarwer DB, Wadden TA, Pertschuk MJ, et al. Body image dissatisfaction and body dysmorphic disorder in 100 cosmetic surgery patients. Plast Reconstr Surg 1998;101:1644–9.
10. Sarwer DB, Cash TF, Magee L, et al. Female college students and cosmetic surgery: an

investigation of experiences, attitudes, and body image. Plast Reconstr Surg 2005;115:931–8.

11. Sperry S, Thompson JK, Sarwer DB, et al. Cosmetic surgery reality TV viewership: relations with cosmetic surgery attitudes, body image and disordered eating. Ann Plast Surg 2009;62:7–11.

12. Henderson-King D, Henderson-King E. Acceptance of cosmetic surgery: scale development and validation. Body Image 2005;2:137–49.

13. Didie ER, Sarwer DB. Factors that influence the decision to undergo cosmetic breast augmentation surgery. J Womens Health 2003;12:241–53.

14. Pertschuk MJ, Sarwer DB, Wadden TA, et al. Body image dissatisfaction in male cosmetic surgery patients. Aesthetic Plast Surg 1998;22:20–4.

15. Sarwer DB, Whitaker LA, Wadden TA, et al. Body image dissatisfaction in women seeking rhytidectomy or blepharoplasty. Aesthetic Surg J 1997;17: 230–4.

16. Sarwer DB, LaRossa D, Bartlett S, et al. Body image concerns of breast augmentation patients. Plast Reconstr Surg 2003;112:83–90.

17. Sarwer DB, Infield AL, Baker JL, et al. Two-year results of a prospective, multi-site investigation of patient satisfaction and psychosocial status following cosmetic surgery. Aesthet Surg J 2008; 28:245–50.

18. Murphy DK, Beckstrand M, Sarwer DB. A prospective multi-center study of psychosocial outcomes after augmentation with natrelle silicone-filled breast implants. Ann Plast Surg 2009;62:118–21.

19. Banbury J, Yetman R, Lucas A, et al. Prospective analysis of the outcome of subpectoral breast augmentation: sensory changes, muscle function, and body image. Plast Reconstr Surg 2004;113: 701–7.

20. Bolton MA, Pruzinsky T, Cash TF, et al. Measuring outcomes in plastic surgery: body image and quality of life in abdominoplasty patients. Plast Reconstr Surg 2003;112:619–25.

21. Cash TF, Duel LA, Perkins LL. Women's psychosocial outcomes of breast augmentation with silicone gel-filled implants: a 2-year prospective study. Plast Reconstr Surg 2002;109:2112–21.

22. Dunofsky M. Psychological characteristics of women who undergo single and multiple cosmetic surgeries. Ann Plast Surg 1997;39:223–8.

23. Sarwer DB, Wadden TA, Whitaker LA. An investigation of changes in body image following cosmetic surgery. Plast Reconstr Surg 2002;109:363–9.

24. Sarwer DB, Magee L. Physical appearance and society. In: Sarwer DB, Pruzinsky T, Cash TF, et al, editors. Psychological aspects of reconstructive and cosmetic plastic surgery: clinical, empirical and ethical perspectives. Philadelphia: Lippincott Williams & Wilkins; 2006. p. 23–36.

25. Phillips KA, McElroy SL, Hudson JI, et al. Body dysmorphic disorder: an obsessive-compulsive spectrum disorder, a form of affective spectrum disorder, or both? J Clin Psychiatry 1995;56:41–51.

26. American Psychiatric Association. Diagnostic and statistical manual of mental disorders. Text Revision. 4th edition. Washington, DC: American Psychiatric Association; 2000.

27. Phillips KA, McElroy SL, Keck PE Jr, et al. A comparison of delusional and nondelusional body dysmorphic disorder in 100 cases. Psychopharmacol Bull 1994;30:179–86.

28. Grant JE, Kim SW, Crow SJ. Prevalence and clinical features of body dysmorphic disorder in adolescent and adult psychiatric inpatients. J Clin Psychiatry 2001;62:517–22.

29. Phillips KA, McElroy SL, Keck PE, et al. Body dysmorphic disorder: 30 cases of imagined ugliness. Am J Psychiatry 1993;150:302–8.

30. Zimmerman M, Mattia JI. Body dysmorphic disorder in psychiatric outpatients: recognition, prevalence, comorbidity, demographic, and clinical correlates. Compr Psychiatry 1998;39:265–70.

31. Sarwer DB, Crerand CE, Didie ER. Body dysmorphic disorder in cosmetic surgery patients. Facial Plast Surg 2003;19:7–17.

32. Bowe WP, Leyden JJ, Crerand CE, et al. Body dysmorphic disorder symptoms among patients with acne vulgaris. J Am Acad Dermatol 2007;57: 222–30.

33. Dufresne RG, Phillips KA, Vittorio CC, et al. A screening questionnaire for body dysmorphic disorder in a cosmetic dermatologic surgery practice. Dermatol Surg 2001;27:457–62.

34. Castle DJ, Phillips KA, Dufresne RG Jr. Body dysmorphic disorder and cosmetic dermatology: more than skin deep. J Cosmet Dermatol 2004;3: 99–103.

35. Crerand CE, Sarwer DB, Magee L, et al. Rate of body dysmorphic disorder among patients seeking facial plastic surgery. Psychiatr Ann 2004;34: 958–65.

36. Vulink NC, Rosenberg A, Plooij JM, et al. Body dysmorphic disorder screening in maxillofacial outpatients presenting for orthognathic surgery. Int J Oral Maxillofac Surg 2008;37:985–91.

37. Hepburn S, Cunningham S. Body dysmorphic disorder in adult orthodontic patients. Am J Orthod Dentofacial Orthop 2006;130:569–74.

38. Cunningham SJ, Bryant CJ, Manisali M, et al. Dysmorphophobia: recent developments of interest to the maxillofacial surgeon. Br J Oral Maxillofac Surg 1996;34:368–74.

39. Cunningham SJ, Feinmann C. Psychological assessment of patients requesting orthognathic surgery and the relevance of body dysmorphic disorder. Br J Orthod 1998;25:293–8.

40. Rispoli A, Acocella A, Pavone I, et al. Psychoemotional assessment changes in patients treated with orthognathic surgery: pre and postsurgery report. World J Orthod 2004;5:48–53.

41. Sarwer DB, Pertschuk MJ, Wadden TA, et al. Psychological investigations in cosmetic surgery: a look back and a look ahead. Plast Reconstr Surg 1998;101:1136–42.

42. Phillips KA, Castle DJ. Body dysmorphic disorder. In: Castle DJ, Phillips KA, editors. Disorders of body image. Hampshire (England): Wrighton Biomedical Publishing; 2002. p. 101–20.

43. Deckersbach T, Savage CR, Phillips KA, et al. Characteristics of memory dysfunction in body dysmorphic disorder. J Int Neuropsychol Soc 2000;6:673–81.

44. Feusner JD, Townsend J, Bystritsky A, et al. Visual information processing of faces in body dysmorphic disorder. Arch Gen Psychiatry 2007;64: 1417–25.

45. Hadley SJ, Newcorn JH, Hollander E. Body dysmorphic disorder: neurobiology and psychopharmacology. In: Castle DJ, Phillips KA, editors. Disorders of body image. Hampshire (England): Wrighton Biomedical Publishing; 2002. p. 139–55.

46. Carey P, Seedat S, Warwick J, et al. SPECT imaging of body dysmorphic disorder. J Neuropsychiatry Clin Neurosci 2004;16:357–9.

47. Feusner JD, Moody T, Hembacher E, et al. Abnormalities of visual processing and frontostriatal systems in body dysmorphic disorder. Arch Gen Psychiatry 2010;67(2):197–205.

48. Phillips KA, Menard W, Fay C, et al. Demographic characteristics, phenomenology, comorbidity, and family history in 200 individuals with body dysmorphic disorder. Psychosomatics 2005;46:317–25.

49. Bienvenu OJ, Samuels JF, Riddle MA, et al. The relationship of obsessive-compulsive disorder to possible spectrum disorders: results from a family study. Biol Psychiatry 2000;48:287–93.

50. Veale D. Advances in a cognitive-behavioural model of body dysmorphic disorder. Body Image 2004;1:113–25.

51. Buhlmann U, Wilhelm S. Cognitive factors in body dysmorphic disorder. Psychiatr Ann 2004;34: 922–6.

52. Phillips KA, Grant JE, Siniscalchi J, et al. Surgical and nonpsychiatric medical treatment of patients with body dysmorphic disorder. Psychosomatics 2001;42:504–10.

53. Kittler JE, Menard W, Phillips KA. Weight concerns in individuals with body dysmorphic disorder. Eat Behav 2007;8:115–20.

54. Phillips KA. The broken mirror. New York: Oxford University Press; 1996.

55. Hollander E, Cohen L, Simeon D. Body dysmorphic disorder. Psychiatr Ann 1993;23:359–64.

56. Rosen JC, Reiter J, Orosan P. Cognitive-behavioral body image therapy for body dysmorphic disorder. J Consult Clin Psychol 1995;63:263–9.

57. Veale D. Outcome of cosmetic surgery and 'DIY' surgery in patients with body dysmorphic disorder. Psychiatr Bull R Coll Psychiatr 2000;24:218.

58. Phillips KA, Diaz SF. Gender differences in body dysmorphic disorder. J Nerv Ment Dis 1997;185: 570–7.

59. Phillips KA, Taub SL. Skin picking as a symptom of body dysmorphic disorder. Psychopharmacol Bull 1995;31:279–88.

60. Veale D, Gournay K, Dryden W, et al. Body dysmorphic disorder: a cognitive behavioural model and pilot randomised controlled trial. Behav Res Ther 1996;34:717–29.

61. Perugi G, Akiskal HS, Giannotti D, et al. Gender-related differences in body dysmorphic disorder. J Nerv Ment Dis 1997;185:570–7.

62. Lucas P. Body dysmorphic disorder and violence: case report and literature review. J Forensic Psychiatr 2002;13:145–56.

63. Albertini R, Phillips KA. Thirty-three cases of body dysmorphic disorder in children and adolescents. J Am Acad Child Adolesc Psychiatry 1999;38: 453–9.

64. Phillips KA, Menard W, Fay C, et al. Psychosocial functioning and quality of life in body dysmorphic disorder. Compr Psychiatry 2005;46:254–60.

65. Buhlmann U, Cook LM, Fama JM, et al. Perceived teasing experiences in body dysmorphic disorder. Body Image 2007;4:381–5.

66. Heinberg LJ. Theories of body image disturbance. In: Thompson JK, editor. Body image, eating disorders and obesity. Washington, DC: American Psychological Association; 1996. p. 27–47.

67. Ishigooka J, Iwao M, Suzuki M, et al. Demographic features of patients seeking cosmetic surgery. Psychiatry Clin Neurosci 1998;52:283–7.

68. Gunstad J, Phillips KA. Axis I comorbidity in body dysmorphic disorder. Compr Psychiatry 2003;44: 270–6.

69. Grant JE, Menard W, Phillips KA. Pathological skin picking in individuals with body dysmorphic disorder. Gen Hosp Psychiatry 2006;28:487–93.

70. Gabbay V, Asnis GM, Bello JA, et al. New onset of body dysmorphic disorder following frontotemporal lesion. Neurology 2003;61:123–5.

71. Phillips KA, McElroy S. Personality disorders and traits in patients with body dysmorphic disorder. Compr Psychiatry 2000;41:229–36.

72. Neziroglu F, McKay D, Todaro J, et al. Effect of cognitive behavior therapy on persons with body dysmorphic disorder and comorbid Axis II diagnoses. Behav Ther 1996;27:67–77.

73. Faravelli C, Salvatori S, Galassi F, et al. Epidemiology of somatoform disorders: a community

survey in Florence. Soc Psychiatry Psychiatr Epidemiol 1997;32:24–9.

74. Otto MW, Wilhelm S, Cohen LS, et al. Prevalence of body dysmorphic disorder in a community sample of women. Am J Psychiatry 2001;158:2061–3.

75. Rief W, Buhlmann U, Wilhelm S, et al. The prevalence of body dysmorphic disorder: a population-based survey. Psychol Med 2006;36:877–85.

76. Mayville S, Katz RC, Gipson MT, et al. Assessing the prevalence of body dysmorphic disorder in an ethnically diverse group of adolescents. J Child Fam Stud 1999;8:357.

77. Bohne A, Keuthen NJ, Wilhelm S, et al. Prevalence of symptoms of body dysmorphic disorder and its correlates: a cross-cultural comparison. Psychosomatics 2002;43:486–90.

78. Bohne A, Wilhelm S, Keuthen NJ, et al. Prevalence of body dysmorphic disorder in a German college student sample. Psychiatry Res 2002;109:101–4.

79. Cansever A, Uzun O, Donmez E, et al. The prevalence and clinical features of body dysmorphic disorder in college students: a study in a Turkish sample. Compr Psychiatry 2003;44:60–4.

80. Biby EL. The relationship between body dysmorphic disorder and depression, self-esteem, somatization, and obsessive-compulsive disorder. J Clin Psychol 1998;54:489–99.

81. Sarwer DB, Whitaker LA, Pertschuk MJ, et al. Body image concerns of reconstructive surgery patients: an under-recognized problem. Ann Plast Surg 1998;40:404–7.

82. De Jongh A, Adair P. Mental disorders in dental practice: a case report of body dysmorphic disorder. Spec Care Dentist 2004;24:61–4.

83. Herren C, Armentrout T, Higgins M. Body dysmorphic disorder: diagnosis and treatment. Gen Dent 2003;51:164–6.

84. Vargel S, Ulusahin A. Psychopathology and body image in cosmetic surgery patients. Aesthetic Plast Surg 2001;25:474–8.

85. Vindigni V, Pavan C, Semenzin M, et al. The importance of recognizing body dysmorphic disorder in cosmetic surgery patients: do our patients need a preoperative psychiatric evaluation? Eur J Plast Surg 2002;25:305–8.

86. Altamura C, Paluello MM, Mundo E, et al. Clinical and subclinical body dysmorphic disorder. Eur Arch Psychiatry Clin Neurosci 2001;251:105–8.

87. Aouizerate B, Pujol H, Grabot D, et al. Body dysmorphic disorder in a sample of cosmetic surgery applicants. Eur Psychiatry 2003;18:365–8.

88. Bellino S, Zizza M, Paradiso E, et al. Dysmorphic concern symptoms and personality disorders: a clinical investigation in patients seeking cosmetic surgery. Psychiatry Res 2006;144:73–8.

89. Vulink NC, Sigurdsson V, Kon M, et al. [Body dysmorphic disorder in 3-8% of patients in outpatient dermatology and plastic surgery clinics]. Ned Tijdschr Geneeskd 2006;150:97–100 [in Dutch].

90. Veale D, De Haro L, Lambrou C. Cosmetic rhinoplasty in body dysmorphic disorder. Br J Plast Surg 2003;56:546–51.

91. Castle DJ, Molton M, Hoffman K, et al. Correlates of dysmorphic concern in people seeking cosmetic enhancement. Aust N Z J Psychiatry 2004;38:439–44.

92. Uzun O, Başoğlu C, Akar A, et al. Body dysmorphic disorder in patients with acne. Compr Psychiatry 2003;44:415–9.

93. Crerand CE, Phillips KA, Menard W, et al. Nonpsychiatric medical treatment of body dysmorphic disorder. Psychosomatics 2005;46:549–55.

94. Phillips KA, Dufresne RG, Wilkel C, et al. Rate of body dysmorphic disorder in dermatology patients. J Am Acad Dermatol 2000;42:436–41.

95. Honigman RJ, Phillips KA, Castle DJ. A review of psychosocial outcomes for patients seeking cosmetic surgery. Plast Reconstr Surg 2004;113:1229–37.

96. Sarwer DB. Psychological assessment of cosmetic surgery patients. In: Sarwer DB, Pruzinsky T, Cash TF, et al, editors. Psychological aspects of reconstructive and cosmetic plastic surgery: clinical, empirical and ethical perspectives. Philadelphia: Lippincott Williams & Wilkins; 2006. p. 267–83.

97. Gorney M. Professional and legal considerations in cosmetic surgery. In: Sarwer DB, Pruzinsky T, Cash TF, et al, editors. Psychological aspects of reconstructive and cosmetic plastic surgery: clinical, empirical and ethical perspectives. Philadelphia: Lippincott Williams & Wilkins; 2006. p. 315–27.

98. Sarwer DB. Awareness and identification of body dysmorphic disorder by aesthetic surgeons: results of a survey of American Society for Aesthetic Plastic Surgery members. Aesthet Surg J 2002;22:531–5.

99. Cotterill JA. Body dysmorphic disorder. Dermatol Clin 1996;14:457–63.

100. Goin JM, Goin MK. Changing the body: psychological effects of plastic surgery. Baltimore (MD): Williams & Wilkens; 1981.

101. Hollander E, Liebowitz M, Winchel R, et al. Treatment of body dysmorphic disorder with serotonin reuptake blockers. Am J Psychiatry 1989;146:768–70.

102. Perugi G, Giannotti D, Di Vaio S, et al. Fluvoxamine in the treatment of the body dysmorphic disorder (dysmorphophobia). Int Clin Psychopharmacol 1996;11:247–54.

103. Phillips KA. Body dysmorphic disorder: clinical aspects and treatment strategies. Bull Menninger Clin 1998;62:A33–48.

104. Phillips KA, Albertini RS, Siniscalchi JM, et al. Effectiveness of pharmacotherapy for body dysmorphic disorder: a chart review study. J Clin Psychiatry 2001;62:721–7.

105. Phillips KA, Dwight MM, McElroy SL. Efficacy and safety of fluvoxamine in body dysmorphic disorder. J Clin Psychiatry 1998;59:165–71.

106. Phillips KA, Najjar F. An open-label study of citalopram in body dysmorphic disorder. J Clin Psychiatry 2003;64:715–20.

107. Hollander E, Allen A, Kwon J, et al. Clomipramine vs. desipramine crossover trial in body dysmorphic disorder. Arch Gen Psychiatry 1999;56:1033–9.

108. Phillips KA, Albertini RS, Rasmussen SA. A randomized placebo-controlled trial of fluoxetine in body dysmorphic disorder. Arch Gen Psychiatry 2002;59:381–8.

109. Nardi AE, Lopes FL, Valenca AM. Body dysmorphic disorder treated with buproprion: case report. Aust N Z J Psychiatry 2005;39:112.

110. Neziroglu FA, Yaryura-Tobias JA. Exposure, response prevention, and cognitive therapy in the treatment of body dysmorphic disorder. Behav Ther 1993;24:431–8.

111. Wilhelm S, Otto M, Zucker B, et al. Prevalence of body dysmorphic disorder in patients with anxiety disorders. J Anxiety Disord 1997;11:499–502.

112. Looper KJ, Kirmayer LJ. Behavioral medicine approaches to somatoform disorders. J Consult Clin Psychol 2002;70:810–27.

113. Williams J, Hadjistavropoulos T, Sharpe D. A meta-analysis of psychological and pharmacological treatments for body dysmorphic disorder. Behav Res Ther 2006;44:99–111.

114. Grossbart TA, Sarwer DB. Psychosocial issues and their relevance to the cosmetic surgery patient. In: Kaminer M, Dover J, Arndt K, editors. Atlas of cosmetic surgery. Philadelphia: WB Saunders; 2001. p. 60–70.

115. Sarwer DB. Psychological considerations in cosmetic surgery. In: Goldwyn RM, Cohen MN, editors. The unfavorable result in plastic surgery. Philadelphia: Lippincott Williams Wilkens; 2001. p. 14–23.

Personality Disorders in Patients Seeking Appearance-Altering Procedures

Jenev Caddell, PsyD[a],*, Jennifer Lyne, MA[b,c]

KEYWORDS

- Obsessive-compulsive personality disorder • Psychological
- Paranoid • Narcissistic

Psychological risk assessment (PRA) is an integral aspect of any clinician's screening process for prospective patients seeking elective appearance-altering procedures (AAPs). One psychological area of concern that may be elusive to the surgeon or even the mental health clinician is a patient's underlying personality disorder. The association between adverse psychological outcomes following AAPs and personality disorders has been documented in the literature.[1–3] This article provides some background regarding psychological risk factors associated with personality disorders for patients seeking AAPs. In addition, the article also provides a brief introduction to personality disorders so that the surgeon may be better prepared to identify these conditions while conducting a PRA.

How to efficiently and accurately screen for psychological risk factors remains unclear. There is a dearth of scientific data to guide predictions of who will fare poorly after cosmetic procedures.[4] It was once thought that screening for psychopathology alone would assist surgeons in determining psychological risk factors, but this process of identification has not proven to be very helpful.[5] Some investigators point out that ideally a full psychological assessment would be done for all patients,[6,7] but clearly, this is not practical. Among the risk factors that might be identified in this process, the one of critical significance is the presence of a personality disorder.

Inside and outside of psychiatry, personality affects all doctor-patient relationships. Davison[8] noted the relevance of personality to all kinds of treatment because it affects help-seeking behaviors, compliance with treatment, coping styles, risk taking, lifestyle choices, and social support, among other elements affecting prognosis and treatment of physical and mental disorders. Moreover, it has been observed that the likelihood of being a "problematic medical patient" is elevated in individuals with personality disorders. This observation underscores the importance of being able to identify these conditions across all medical settings.[9]

In a review of the literature on psychosocial outcomes for patients seeking cosmetic surgery, Honigman and colleagues[4] found that having a personality disorder was one among the major risk factors associated with poor outcome. Although perhaps outdated, one study of psychological disturbance following otherwise successful surgery found that 50% of patients were diagnosed with a personality disorder.[10] In another study, narcissistic personality disorder was found to be one factor adversely affecting the outcome for some patients.[11] Given the prevalence of personality disorders among patients seeking

a Private Practice, 1133 Broadway, Suite 1028, New York, NY 10010, USA
b Clinical Psychology Program, Fairleigh Dickinson University, 1000 River Road, Teaneck, NJ 07666, USA
c Interpersonal Communications Laboratory, Department of Communication Sciences, Child Psychiatry, New York Psychiatric Institute, 1051 Riverside Drive, New York, NY 10032, USA
* Corresponding author.
E-mail address: jenev@drjenevcaddell.com

Oral Maxillofacial Surg Clin N Am 22 (2010) 455–460
doi:10.1016/j.coms.2010.07.003

cosmetic surgery and other AAPs as well as the amplification of psychological risk for a patient who has a personality disorder, it is particularly important for the surgeon to be aware of these conditions and to have some kind of basis for their detection.

According to the *Diagnostic and Statistical Manual of Mental Disorders, Fourth Edition, Text Revision* (DSM-IV-TR), a personality disorder is defined as "an enduring pattern of inner experiences and behavior that deviates markedly from the expectations of the individual's culture. This pattern is manifested in two or more of the following areas: cognition (ie, ways of perceiving and interpreting self, other people and events); affectivity (ie, the range, intensity, lability, and appropriateness of emotional response); interpersonal functioning and impulse control."[12(p686)] To diagnose a personality disorder, the pattern must be rigid and pervasive in multiple if not all areas of the person's life. Like most disorders, for a diagnosis to be made, the pattern must lead to clinically significant distress or impairment in occupational, social, or other significant areas of functioning in life.

This DSM-IV-TR definition should not be considered the only way of describing all of the personality disorder symptoms that might be of concern to clinicians because mental health clinicians' ideas about personality disorders seem to vary. According to Shedler and Westen,[13(p1350)] "a clinically useful and empirically sound classification of personality disorders has been an elusive ideal." Diagnosis is further complicated because these patients frequently have more than 1 personality disorder. In addition, psychologists and psychiatrists often report patients presenting with certain features of a personality disorder that are not captured by the diagnostic criteria set forth by the DSM-IV-TR. One study indicates that 86.5% of the surveyed clinicians at Harvard Medical School treated patients with a variety of neurotic personality symptoms but did not formally categorize them as having personality disorders.[14]

There are also problems with the assessment of personality disorders. This assessment is typically deferred in mental heath settings until the clinician has spent considerable time with the patient. When personality disorders must be diagnosed more quickly, self-report measures are used, which can be problematic because individuals with personality disorders frequently have little or no insight into their disorder and are unable to report symptoms. These patients often think that the interpersonal problems they experience are the fault of others. These patients may also be deceptive or so concerned with the impression they give that they will exaggerate strengths or deny weaknesses. Validity data are therefore much weaker for self-report measures of personality disorders than for other clinical disorders.[15]

It is also important to recognize that the number of people with personality disorders in a variety of medical settings is often underestimated. For example, Casey and Tyrer[16] have reported that up to one-third of patients seen by primary care physicians meet diagnostic criteria for a personality disorder. These disorders are also common in mental health settings but are much less often the focus of treatment than are comorbid disorders such as major depressive disorder or bipolar disorder.[8]

In a national survey of more than 1800 psychiatrists and psychologists, Westen[14] tried to determine which techniques are used by most mental health professionals in their diagnosis of personality disorders. Clinicians surveyed indicated that in their diagnosis of a personality disorder, they rely on their own inferences after hearing patients' narratives about their lives and relationships and also pay attention to their observations about patients' behaviors toward them during the interview rather than rely on direct diagnostic questions or assessment instruments.

It is apparent that specialists in mental health such as psychologists and psychiatrists have difficulties with the definition of a personality disorder put forth by the DSM-IV-TR, and there is no clear and efficient method to quickly screen for these disorders. Surely then, it is problematic for clinicians performing AAPs, who have less training and experience in the study of personality, to determine which of their patients meet the criteria for a personality disorder. It is agreed, however, that attention to patients' behavior as well as a sensitive and careful listening to their narratives are imperative elements of any screening process for personality disorders.

Despite the limitations noted earlier, it is important for oral and maxillofacial surgeons and others performing AAPs to be acquainted with the definitions and common characteristics of personality disorders and to be wary of those likely to be associated with an adverse outcome.

PERSONALITY DISORDERS: A SUMMARY

The DSM-IV-TR groups personality disorders into 3 major categories or clusters. Cluster A contains personality patterns that are considered odd or eccentric, with emotional withdrawal, including paranoid, schizoid, and schizotypal personality disorders. Cluster B is composed of the disorders in which people present with dramatic or exaggerated emotionality, including antisocial, borderline, histrionic, and narcissistic personality disorders. Cluster C includes the disorders in which the presentation is anxious and characterized by resistive submissiveness, including avoidant, dependent, and obsessive-compulsive personality disorders. Each of these disorders is presented with a description of how a patient who has this disorder might present.

CLUSTER A

Cluster A includes 3 personality disorders: paranoid, schizoid, and schizotypal. None of these disorders are particularly likely to be present in patients seeking AAPs, so they are discussed only briefly.

Millon,[17(p695)] a renowned expert on the presentation and assessment of personality disorders, describes the paranoid personality as one that has its origins in lack of basic trust in others: "There is evidence that in many cases the paranoid person has received sadistic treatment during early infancy. Due to his lack of trust, he must be vigilant in order to safeguard himself against sudden deception and attack, and is exquisitely sensitive to traces of hostility, contempt, criticism or accusation." Although not particularly inclined to seek AAPs, patients with paranoid personality are of concern to clinicians because of their tendency to be unforgiving, hostile, and litigious, with retaliations based on the perceptions of having been wronged. During the interview, these patients may feel interrogated and react defensively by questioning the clinician's line of inquiry.

Also not particularly inclined to seek cosmetic procedures, the schizoid personality "lacks the ability to experience the joyful and pleasurable aspects in life."[17(p217)] The typical presentation of the schizoid personality is one of extreme emotional distance, introversion, and detachment. Questions about the patient's relationships with others are important because the person with this personality disorder is likely to be socially isolated, neither desiring nor enjoying any kind of relationships with others, including sexual relationships. Schizoid personality is marked by the seeming absence of any kind of emotionality, and it is extremely difficult, if not impossible, to establish a rapport with someone who has this disorder.

Perhaps the least motivated to seek AAPs may be the person with schizotypal personality disorder, who is quite similar to someone with schizophrenia. Millon[17(p613)] describes the schizotypal personality thus: "Manifest in the schizotypal personality are a variety of persistent and prominent eccentricities of behavior, thought and perception, which mirrors, but falls short of the features that would justify the diagnosis of schizophrenia." The presentation is somewhat odd or eccentric, with inappropriate or constricted affect, possibly unique clothing, and a strange sense of humor. Affect at times can be intense, with lasting eye contact when patients are discussing a topic in which they are invested. Patients with schizotypal personality disorder are much more interested than those with schizoid personality disorder, and rapport is more easily established if the clinician is careful not to be judging or rejecting. Individuals with schizotypal personality disorder may also present with paranoia or ideas of reference (eg, the television or radio is talking directly to them).

CLUSTER B

Cluster B disorders include antisocial, borderline, histrionic, and narcissistic personality disorders and are known as the dramatic, emotional, or erratic disorders. Unlike the coldness of the patients with Cluster A disorders, those with Cluster B disorders typically present as colorful or exaggerated, but beneath their dramatic display, it is often difficult to get a true sense of their inner life. These individuals have ample capacity to experience pleasure and enhance their lives, albeit in an unbalanced way, typically by being either too self-inclined or too inclined toward others.[17(p325)] However, the capacity of such individuals to seek pleasure and enhancement makes them likely candidates for AAPs.

The hallmark of histrionic personality disorder is an overly gregarious presentation with an exaggerated but shallow sense of emotionality. People with histrionic personality disorder are dependent on admiration and affection, and their center of gravity lies in others, not in themselves. "Histrionic personalities are active, they do not sit passively waiting for the competence, and skills of others to give shape to their lives. They do not cling or seek nurturance. Rather, the principal goal is securing attention and approval as a means to avoid disinterest or abandonment."[17(p325)] These people often dress in attention-grabbing clothing and are likely to behave charmingly or seductively while being interviewed, whereas underneath the dramatic flair and liveliness, questions are often answered vaguely and without details. It can be difficult to get a precise answer, and histrionic patients may exaggerate physical symptoms for the sake of getting attention. Approval and attention are central to their sense of identity, which is often overly dependent on their appearance and as such may lead to unrealistic expectations of the results from cosmetic surgery and other AAPs.

Antisocial personality disorder is characterized by the disregard for and violation of the rights of others. People with antisocial personality disorder are sometimes referred to as sociopaths and are noted to have no remorse or empathy for others. This disorder is more commonly diagnosed in men than in women. Of note, these people possess a "superficial charm" and can be manipulative and exploitative. People with antisocial personality disorder have low frustration tolerance, and in an interview, such individuals may easily become angry and critical if one does not submit to their manipulations. People with antisocial personality disorder are more prone to abuse substances and may be aggressive or violent. It is important to ask questions about their previous problems with school or with the law.

Narcissism refers to excessive self-love, and patients with narcissistic personality disorder present with an exceptional self-interest and self-involvement. These patients are notorious for their sense of grandiosity, entitlement, and inflated sense of self-importance and tend to have unreasonable demands of favorable treatment, lack empathy for others, and frequently take advantage of others to pursue their own selfish goals. Underneath this front of grandiosity is generally an individual who is fragile and insecure and may react to criticism with rage, shame, or humiliation, as though his or her sense of self-worth is as fragile as a house of cards. Renowned psychotherapist, Otto Kernberg, describes this personality type:

Narcissistic patients present an unusual degree of self-reference in their interactions with other people, a great need to be loved and admired by others, and a curious apparent contradiction between a very inflated concept of themselves and an inordinate need for tribute from others. Their emotional life is shallow. They experience little empathy for the feelings of others, they obtain very little enjoyment from life other than from the tributes they receive from others or from their own grandiose fantasies, and they feel restless and bored when external glitter wears off and no new sources feed their self-regard. They envy others, tend to idealize some people from whom they expect narcissistic supplies, and to depreciate and treat with contempt those from whom they do not expect anything (often their former idols). In general, their relationships with other people are clearly exploitative and sometimes parasitic. It is as if they feel they have the right to control and possess others and to exploit them without guilt feelings—and behind a surface which very often is charming and engaging, one senses coldness and ruthlessness. Very often such patients are considered to be 'dependent' because they need so much tribute and adoration from others, but on a deeper level they are completely unable really to depend on anybody because of their deep distrust and depreciation of others.[17(p655)]

Clinicians performing AAPs should be wary of patients with narcissistic personality disorder. These individuals are likely to have unrealistic expectations of results, a fragile sense of self that is dependent on looks and easily shattered, and a sense of entitlement that could lead to litigation.

The last Cluster B diagnosis is borderline personality disorder, so called because patients were thought to be somewhere on the continuum between neurosis and psychosis. Borderline personality disorder is an advanced and potentially serious level of maladaptive personality dysfunctions, with the most salient feature being the extreme depth and variability of moods. According to Millon,[17(p646)] "Borderlines tend to experience extended periods of dejection and disillusionment interspersed with brief excursions of euphoria, and significantly more frequent episodes of irritability, self-destructive acts, and impulsive anger. These moods are often unpredictable and appear prompted less by external events than internal factors." Patients with borderline personality disorder often complain of chronic emptiness and have intense fear of abandonment, misinterpreting the behaviors of others as indicating rejection, which can lead to suicidality as well as less serious but still concerning acts of self-mutilation, including cutting. These patients tend to oscillate between idealization and devaluation of others. A first indication of borderline personality disorder in patients is the overly complimentary nature, indicating that their physician is the best they have ever met, whereas previous physicians and/or people in their life have been truly despicable. Inevitably, the new physician, too, will be placed in the latter group for some innocuous slight, and these well-related and charming patients will return full of criticism, rage, and even violence toward their physician. Millon[17(p655)] discusses the causes of this all-good or all-bad appraisal of others: "There is a morbid fear of abandonment and a wish for protective nurturance, preferably received by constant physical proximity to the rescuer. The baseline position is friendly dependency on a nurturer, which becomes hostile control if the caregiver or lover fails to deliver enough (and there is never enough)." Clearly, clinicians must proceed very carefully when they suspect that a patient may have borderline personality disorder and respectfully require an outside psychiatric evaluation.

CLUSTER C

Cluster C personality diagnoses include the avoidant, dependent, and obsessive-compulsive personality disorders. Cluster C groups together disorders that share a sense of anxiety and resistive submissiveness, and people with these personality disorders frequently present as tense and worried. These people may seem quite controlled and cautious as well as concerned with a clinician's assessment of them.

People with avoidant personality show an excessive preoccupation and oversensitivity to the stresses of life, such that they invest all of their energy avoiding pain and misfortune.[17(p217)] People with avoidant personality disorder are more socially isolated because of their hypersensitivity to criticism or rejection. During an interview, patients who are avoidant may seem to be withdrawn, vague, suspicious, or anxious. Once trust is established, with empathic and sensitive questioning that patients do not mistake as criticism, patients with avoidant personality disorder are generally able to discuss their fears of rejection. These patients generally desire close relationships, unlike those with schizoid personality disorder of Cluster A, but are too fearful to enter into one. It is especially important to establish an atmosphere of understanding in patients with personality disorder so that their motivation for surgery can be safely explored. Patients whose motivation is for secondary gain (ie, "I want a nicer nose so that I can get a boyfriend") rather than for primary gain (ie, "I have always hated my huge ugly nose and I am tired of looking at it") present much greater risk for the surgeon and are not likely to be good candidates for surgery. This is one reason for carefully exploring the motivations of every patient seeking AAP. Patients with avoidant personality disorder will likely feel comfortable sharing their motivation in a safe and empathic context.

In contrast to patients with paranoid personality disorder, individuals who presents with dependent personality disorder will likely be trusting and deferential. Such individuals will regard the surgeon as an expert and will likely have confidence in the surgeon's recommendations. These patients may have little or no recognition of the lack of initiative in their own lives and generally feel unable to make their own decisions. The clinician might suspect dependent personality disorder by the way the patients easily place their care in the interviewer's hands and put the clinician in charge. If a patient is suspected to have features of this disorder, it is important to determine whether motivation to undergo an AAP is internal or external. This patient may go to great lengths, including tolerating abuse in an effort to maintain a relationship, and has difficulty being alone or voicing opinions. As always, it is critical to learn about important others in the patient's life and determine whether they may play a role in the patient's decision to seek AAP.

The final personality disorder for discussion is obsessive-compulsive personality disorder. Patients with this disorder are so fixated on perfectionism that it is nearly impossible for them to get things done. There is a central focus on details, so much so that everything else seems to be lost. It may be difficult to get to the content of the interview because of the fixation on the details and words themselves. The evaluation process may feel like a struggle and it will be difficult to establish rapport. The person with obsessive-compulsive disorder may have difficulty throwing things away and might have issues of hoarding. Such patients may sacrifice relationships and recreation for a complete devotion to work and are excessively concerned with lists, rules, and order. Emotionally and financially, people with obsessive-compulsive personality disorder are notoriously stingy. Such people have difficulty tolerating mistakes or imperfection, and as might be expected, the trait of obsessiveness was found to be the most frequently noted trait in a study of personality among patients seeking rhinoplasty.[3] The difficulty with control and parsimony may keep many people with obsessive-compulsive personality disorder away from elective surgery, but for those who seek such procedures, it is important that the surgeon is aware of the potential problems. Critical and perfectionist, the outcome of any procedure is likely to be disappointing for the patient with obsessive-compulsive personality disorder, which may lead to litigation.

Although obsessive-compulsive personality disorder is classified as a somatoform disorder in the DSM-IV, body dysmorphic disorder (BDD), formerly known as dysmorphophobia, is probably the psychiatric diagnosis with which plastic surgeons are most familiar. BDD is a psychiatric disorder involving excessive preoccupation with a minimal or imagined defect in one's body. The DSM-IV estimates a prevalence of 0.7% to 1.1% of BDD in the community.[12] Various investigators have reported that the rate of BDD among candidates seeking plastic surgery is between 7% and 15%.[5,18,19] The literature on the subject indicates that people with BDD often experience psychological adverse outcomes to AAPs, with some patients lashing out even violently toward the treating physician.[20,21] It is important for the surgeon to be aware of the risk factors related to BDD and the methods to effectively screen patients for this disorder.

Several studies have noted the comorbidity of BDD and various personality disorders in patients seeking cosmetic surgery. For example, in a group of 66 patients seeking cosmetic surgery, the severity of dysmorphic symptoms was found to be most significantly related to the number of diagnostic criteria met for both schizotypal and paranoid personality disorders, with significant correlations also with borderline, avoidant, and obsessive-compulsive personality disorders.[1] Clinicians should use extra precaution if they are considering a candidate who might present with BDD or traits associated with any of the earlier-mentioned personality disorders.

The practice of PRA is an indispensable component of the screening process for patients seeking elective AAPs. Despite the need for more literature in PRA, some risk factors for psychological adverse outcomes have been established. Among these risk factors are personality disorders, which have been reviewed in this article. Although a suspected personality disorder should not disqualify a prospective patient, it is among the conditions suggesting that the clinician should proceed with caution. It is highly recommended that any doubt about the psychological health of a patient seeking AAP should prompt the clinician to consult with a mental health professional. When appropriate, clinicians should consider referring prospective patients for a more complete psychological evaluation before deciding to proceed with elective AAP.

REFERENCES

1. Bellino S, Zaizza M, Paradiso E, et al. Dysmorphic concern symptoms and personality disorders: a clinical investigation in patients seeking cosmetic surgery. Psychiatry Res 2006;144:73–8.

2. Napolean A. The presentation of personalities in plastic surgery. Ann Plast Surg 1993;31:286–7.

3. Zojaji R, Javanbakht M, Ghanadan A, et al. High prevalence of personality abnormalities in patients seeking rhinoplasty. Otolaryngol Head Neck Surg 2007;137:83–7.

4. Honigman RJ, Phillips KA, Castle DJ. A review of psychosocial outcomes for patients seeking cosmetic surgery. Plast Reconstr Surg 2004;113:1229–37.

5. Sarwer DB, Pertschuk MJ, Wadden TA, et al. Psychological investigation in cosmetic surgery: a look back and a look ahead. Plast Reconstr Surg 1998;101:1136–42.

6. Cunningham SJ, Feinmann C. Psychological assessment of patients requesting orthognathic surgery and the relevance of body dysmorphic disorder. Br J Orthod 1998;25:293–8.

7. McLaughlin JK, Wise TN, Lipworth L. Increased risk of suicide among patients with breast implants: do the epidemiologic data support psychiatric consultation? Psychosomatics 2004;45:277–80.

8. Davison SE. Principles of managing patients with personality disorders. Advances in Psychiatric Treatment 2002;8:1–9.

9. Emerson J, Pankratz L, Joos S, et al. Personality disorders in problematic medical patients. Psychosomatics 1994;35:469–73.

10. Edgerton MT, Jacobsen WE, Meyer E. Surgical-psychiatric study of patients seeking plastic (cosmetic) surgery: ninety-eight consecutive patients with minimal deformity. Br J Plast Surg 1960;13:136–43.

11. Wright MR, Wright WK. A psychological study of patients undergoing cosmetic surgery. Arch Otolaryngol 1975;101:145–51.

12. American Psychiatric Association. Diagnostic and statistical manual of mental disorders. Text Revision (DSM-IV-TR). 4th edition. Washington, DC: APA; 2000.

13. Shedler J, Westen D. Refining personality disorder diagnosis: integrating science and practice. Am J Psychiatry 2004;161:1350–65.

14. Westen D. Divergences between clinical and research methods for assessing personality disorders: implications for research and the evolution of axis II. Am J Psychiatry 1997;154:895–903.

15. Westen D, Shedler J. Revising and assessing axis II: part I: developing a clinically and empirically valid assessment measure. Am J Psychiatry 1999;156:258–72.

16. Casey PR, Tyrer P. Personality disorder and psychiatric illness in general medical practice. Br J Psychiatry 1990;156:261–5.

17. Millon T. Disorders of personality: DSM-IV and beyond. 2nd edition. New York: Wiley-Interscience; 1996.

18. Sarwer DB, Wadden TA, Whitaker LA. An investigation of changes in body image following cosmetic surgery. Plast Reconstr Surg 2002;109:363–9.

19. Ishigooka J, Iwao M, Suzuki M, et al. Demographic features of patients seeking cosmetic surgery. Psychiatry Clin Neurosci 1998;52:283–7.

20. Phillips KA, Grant J, Siniscalchi J, et al. Surgical and nonpsychiatric medical treatments of patients with body dysmorphic disorder. Psychosomatics 2001;42:504.

21. Phillips KA, Diaz SF. Gender differences in body dysmorphic disorder. J Nerv Ment Dis 1997;185:570–7.

Management of the Uncooperative Child

Meredith Blitz, DDS[a,b,c,*],
Kate Cerino Britton, MSEd, MA, BCBA[d]

KEYWORDS
- Pediatric • Oral surgery • Mental health • Behavior
- Autism spectrum disorders • Anesthesia

The management of a child who requires a medical procedure is a challenging issue for providers, patients, and families. It is particularly challenging for the oral and maxillofacial surgeon (OMS) and practitioners in the dental specialties. The office of the OMS is traditionally one in which short outpatient procedures are performed within brief appointment times often using only local anesthesia. For typical children, this brief procedure may be difficult, and for children with behavioral challenges, it may be impossible without the use of behavioral management techniques or pharmacologic modalities.

In the past, techniques to manage behaviorally challenged patients were limited, and these patients were often subjected to outpatient general anesthesia to accomplish simple surgical goals. However, with an increasing number of pediatric patients with mild to severe behavioral challenges, alternate approaches must be evaluated, taught, and practiced by clinicians who are involved in the surgical care of children.

In an article published March 19, 2000 in the *New York Times*, a 5-year-old male patient allegedly sustained a femur fracture while being actively restrained by his dentist. Although reports of injury such as this are rare, the management of uncooperative children is an important issue. Practitioners must be aware of current trends in pediatric mental health and should develop treatment protocols to avoid complications.

INCIDENCE

In the *Report of the Surgeon General's Conference on Children's Mental Health: A National Action Agenda* published in 2000, three major Federal Departments, the Department of Health and Human Services, the Department of Education, and the Department of Justice, were brought together to collaborate on a vision and goals for the pediatric population with mental illness. The low priority of this issue and the stigma surrounding mental illness are both factors contributing to the limited access these patients have to education and routine care. This action agenda included and prioritized the following goal, to "train frontline providers to recognize and manage mental health-care issues, and educate mental health providers about scientifically-proven prevention and treatment strategies."[1] To accomplish this goal, the suggested focus was the education and training of medical professionals in all aspects of childhood development and differences; training to enhance practitioners' knowledge base in these areas; development of multidisciplinary programs for health care professionals, which allow for a focus on pediatric mental health; and training support for professionals to keep abreast of new developments in the field of children's mental health.

However, a decade later, most dental schools and residency training programs of oral and

[a] Division of Dentistry, Department of Oral and Maxillofacial Surgery, Seton Hall University, 400 South Orange Avenue, South Orange, NJ 07079-2689, USA
[b] Department of Oral and Maxillofacial Surgery, University of Medicine and Dentistry of New Jersey, 110 Bergen Street, Newark, NJ 07103, USA
[c] Department of Oral and Maxillofacial Surgery, St Joseph's Regional Medical Center, 703 Main Street, Paterson, NJ 07503, USA
[d] Alpine Learning Group, 777 Paramus Road, Paramus, NJ 07652, USA
* Corresponding author. Department of Oral and Maxillofacial Surgery, St Joseph's Regional Medical Center, 703 Main Street, Paterson, NJ 07503.
E-mail address: Blitzgme@umdnj.edu

Oral Maxillofacial Surg Clin N Am 22 (2010) 461–469
doi:10.1016/j.coms.2010.08.002

maxillofacial surgery provide limited education in pediatric behavioral management for the outpatient setting. With the nation facing a public health crisis in mental health care for children and adolescents, almost all practitioners come into contact with a child with mental health problems that interfere with normal development and functioning.

According to the surgeon general's report, "one in ten children and adolescents suffer from mental illness severe enough to cause some level of impairment. Recent evidence compiled by the WHO indicates that by the year 2020, childhood neuropsychiatric disorders will rise proportionately by over 50 percent, internationally, to become one of the five most common causes of morbidity, mortality, and disability among children."[2] With this focus on childhood mental illness and its increasing prevalence, practitioners must stay updated in management strategies to facilitate proper care and positive outcomes in the mentally disabled pediatric patient.

The true incidence of individual mental health disorders in children has been difficult to obtain. Many factors, including concurrent mental health disorders, stigmatization leading to lack of parental admission and diagnosis, lack of access to services including diagnosis, and insurance regulatory issues, have led to difficulties in identifying all individuals in this subset of the population. However, with the recent reported increases in autism spectrum disorders (ASDs), a focus shift is occurring at the ground level and parents and practitioners are encouraged to seek early detection and intervention.

The Centers for Disease Control and Prevention now estimates that ASDs affect approximately 1 in 110 children.[3] ASDs are most commonly known as Asperger disorder, pervasive developmental disorder-not otherwise specified, and autism. Attention deficit disorder (ADD) with or without hyperactivity has been even more challenging to quantify. A recent study revealed a cumulative incidence of attention-deficit/hyperactivity disorder (ADHD) of 7.5%.[4] Additional disorders that are common in children and adolescents include oppositional defiance disorder, Tourette syndrome, anxiety disorders, childhood schizophrenia, aggressive conduct, bipolar disorders, and major depression. Many of the diagnosed children have comorbid conditions and can be categorized by more than one major disorder. This challenge makes the true incidence of each disorder very difficult to quantify. Both the *Diagnostic and Statistical Manual of Mental Disorders* (Fourth Edition) and the *International Statistical Classification of Diseases, Ninth Revision* provide valuable information on the levels to which patients can be affected and on what a true crisis these disorders and others represent.

PREVIOUS TREATMENT STRATEGIES

In the past, many behavioral techniques have been used in an attempt to treat children and facilitate a positive learning experience with successful treatment outcomes. However, when dealing with a surge of patients with behavioral challenges, many of these techniques could become obsolete and potentially lead to future fear and anxiety in relation to oral care.

The technique most commonly used with pediatric patients has been the "tell, show, do" approach to learning. This technique can be very effective because it allows for desensitization to stimuli and a general understanding by the children of what they should expect in the oral care setting. However, many behaviorally challenged children have unusual fears and sensory processing issues along with verbal comprehension difficulties. This technique can be successfully initiated in the home by the child's parents and then transferred to the clinical setting. Should a patient have receptive language delays, this technique may or may not be effective. Many children with ASDs are visual learners, so visual presentation of materials can be helpful. Limited discussion and simple commands work best in this patient population (**Fig. 1**).

Papoose boards for managing children are still used in the dental setting and in hospital

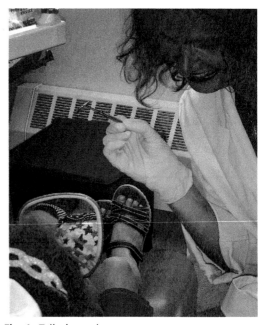

Fig. 1. Tell, show, do.

emergency departments. The papoose is designed to restrain a child in a safe soft fabric on a hard backboard. The child is placed in a supine position and secured into the device with only the head exposed. Without the ability to move the body, simple procedures may be performed without the risk of injury due to flailing or movement. Although effective, this type of device can create anxiety and fear in both the patient and parent. It may be frightening for a child to be restrained so restrictively and also can be a psychological challenge for the parent who must consent to, allow for, and observe their child in this situation. This technique is best used in acute or emergency care only and requires full parental consent. For elective procedures, all attempts should be made to use nonrestraining techniques to achieve care.

Hand-over-mouth technique is designed to regain control of a child who is verbalizing inappropriately or having a tantrum. This technique also requires parental consent and parents who are willing to allow the coverage of the patient's mouth. The practitioner should be cautioned that biting is a concern in aggressive children. However, when applied appropriately, this technique may allow the child to regain composure and focus on instructions from the surgeon and team.

Passive and active manual restraint techniques are still commonly used. Parents are often participants, and at the practitioner's instruction, the staff gently or, if needed, firmly restrain a patient to complete certain aspects of care. This technique has often facilitated local anesthesia administration and limits the child's movements during invasive portions of the procedure. The technique is often tolerated well by patients and parents and allows for the completion of challenging portions of scheduled procedures. However, in the behaviorally challenged group of pediatric patients, aversion to physical touch may make this approach counterproductive. The issue of touch aversion should be discussed before the patient's appointment so that alternate techniques may be assessed for use.

CURRENT MODALITIES/BEHAVIORAL TECHNIQUES

As behavioral therapies become increasingly popular in the school and private settings, it is desirable for OMSs and other clinicians to acquire a basic knowledge of the existence and use of these therapies. This understanding provides clinicians with a background in their function and promotes the application of theses behavioral therapies in the office of the OMS and other medical settings. Behaviorists use various techniques to help challenged children, adolescents, and adults to achieve goals that might not otherwise be obtainable. These techniques are often time consuming and difficult to implement for clinicians untrained in these methods. However, through education and practice, these programs can enhance the practice of an OMS and allow for the successful treatment of individuals with behavioral concerns, particularly the pediatric population.

Social stories interventions are designed to use short stories about specific concepts to facilitate learning in children. These interventions are often used to improve the social skills of children with ASDs but may be implemented with any child, including the uncooperative patient with or without a diagnosis of ASD. Social stories tend to describe a situation in very concrete and simple terms and the associated relevant social cues, perspectives of individuals in the stories, and suggest the patient's appropriate response to the cues in the stories. The effectiveness of these stories is related to the omission of irrelevant information and focus on being descriptive to help the individual understand the basics of the situation and the expectations. There are visual and text portions that help provide cues for accomplishing a task while helping to establish clear socialization cues and responses.

There are published social stories available for the behaviorally challenged child, which relate to visiting the dentist. However, the OMS's setting is different, with invasive treatment almost always necessary, whereas general dental experiences, including examination and hygiene procedures, may be noninvasive in nature. The need for injections and potentially misunderstood painful stimuli may produce anxiety and behavioral outbursts in the OMS's setting. It is up to the treating surgeon to provide a social story that is individualized to patient needs and office visit expectations. The goal of the social story is to help the learner understand the events and expectations so that the new understanding of what is expected leads to improved behavior. Although social stories were introduced in the 1990s, the effectiveness of this behavioral technique has not been researched extensively. Nonetheless, with little, if any, apparent downside to this technique, social stories may be tried on any and all pediatric uncooperative patients.

Video modeling is a form of learning by observation in which desirable behaviors and appropriate responses may be acquired by watching video demonstrations of skills. Individuals, after observation, should then successfully imitate the target behavior. This modality has been used for social skill acquisition, to enhance communication skills, and even in the realm of athletic performance. Video self-modeling is a variation of this technique in which individuals watch themselves successfully perform a behavior and again imitate the behavior repeatedly in an effort to generalize the skill. Video modeling was shown to be effective in older children who were not successful using other therapies for learning.[5]

These interventions have shown promise in the population with ASD. However, these interventions might be applicable to many children before a dental or surgical office visit as a tool to reduce anxiety related to unknown surroundings and events. Videos made by the surgical team can be sent ahead of time to all appointed children. If the child is severely challenged, school personnel can become involved and provide support for the child before and between scheduled visits. Pretreatment videos can be shown to the patient at both home and school. Once children arrive for their scheduled visit, consideration can be made for video self-modeling. The patient may actually want to participate, and this self-modeling can also serve as a distraction or reinforcement of desired behavior. The video can be taken home and reviewed with parents or therapists to focus on the generalization of the skill set.

In the outpatient oral surgery practice, patient flow is often fast paced. The patient is examined, the treatment is planned, and the patient is treated in a limited time frame, typically between 15 and 60 minutes. Children with behavioral disorders may have difficulties in new surroundings and with new people. Although it might be perceived as a waste of time, multiple introductory visits, with stepwise addition of new expectations and procedures, can facilitate a successful interaction and enable the clinician to conduct the necessary treatment. These visits should be kept short, and at each subsequent visit, new expectations can be added and additional tasks performed. Visit success can be measured by data recording and a review of the effectiveness and completion of each step as it is added to the treatment protocol. Although tailored to the general dental environment, **Table 1** provides a simple framework and can be adapted to procedures in the oral surgical environment.

Skill acquisition programming for uncooperative children is an advanced behavioral intervention that is most often used for children with severe obstructions to learning and for tolerating community-based office visits. Skill acquisition programs are most commonly used by advanced specialists in behavior analysis, including Board Certified Behavior Analysts. School and home programming, designed to work with severely affected children, outlines tasks in simple step-by-step instructions. The child starts with the first instruction and advances to each step as success is achieved. Data are collected by the instructor and often charted or graphed for outcomes analysis. Measurable criteria are set before instituting these programs, and when met, the child may move on to the next step. Should the step not be mastered, the child returns to preceding steps or stays on the current step until mastery is achieved (see **Table 1**).

Skill acquisition programs may begin in the home or school with trained therapists and then be introduced in the clinical setting. The professional may be asked to provide equipment necessary to complete the examination before the visit. This style of teaching may be time consuming and may require multiple visits to the office before completion of planned procedures. With more schools and professionals using applied behavioral analysis techniques, the dentist or surgeon may be asked to participate in these trials. A working knowledge of the clinician's role and of appropriate interventions in this patient population allows for timely acquisition of these skills and future generalization.

Preparation for certain issues can be incorporated within skill acquisition programs. When faced with a time count, most children are able to achieve a desired goal. Children with challenges are no different. Counting over a period can be used, and children can be told that for a definitive count, they must complete a portion or a step of the procedure. For example, children can be told that they must maintain an open mouth for a count of 10 for an examination. The count can then be adjusted by counting at a faster or slower pace such that the result still arrives at 10 for the child. This technique may prove to be very effective and may be applicable to each part of the procedure.

Also used and effective in some children are reinforcement systems that allow the child to gain access to a toy, video game, television show, or other desired reward (**Fig. 2**). Reinforcement systems and access to preferred activities and toys must be discussed with the parent or therapist before their use so that the practitioner is appropriately prepared (**Fig. 3**). With the successful completion of each step, the child is allowed access to the desired reinforcing object or activity for a certain period. For example, children who hold their mouth open for the count of 10 during an examination can be given immediate access to a video game of choice and be allowed

Table 1
Tolerates visit to the dentist

Alpine Learning Group, Inc
Task Analysis Data Sheet

Learner's Name: **Criterion:** 90% for 2 consecutive sessions
Program:

Sr+=
EC=

Step	Score each response as follows: (C) correct (I) incorrect (P) prompted
1. Tolerates sitting in chair	
2. Tolerates chair reclining	
3. Opens Wide	
4. Tolerates mirror in mouth	
5. Tolerates mirror in mouth to a count of 10	
6. Tolerates counting teeth with pick	
7. Tolerates counting teeth while pushing and scraping teeth with pick	
8. Tolerates tongue blade in mouth	
9. Tolerates tongue blade in mouth to a count of 10	
10. Tolerates cotton roll in mouth	
11. Tolerates cotton roll in mouth to a count of 10	
12. Tolerates placement of a lead vest over chest	
13. Tolerates wearing a lead vest to a count of 10	
14. Tolerates film in mouth	
15. Tolerates film in mouth to a count of 10	
16. Tolerates non-powered polisher in mouth to a count of 10	
17. Tolerates powered polisher in mouth to a count of 10	
18. Tolerates Mr. Thirsty in mouth to a count of 10	
19. Rinses with Water	
Total:	

to play for a length of time predetermined by the practitioner. This time can be limited to 30 to 60 seconds and repeated with each successful step.

One of the most effective management steps is repetition of skills to secure patient acceptance and future generalization. The goal of many of these techniques is to allow for comfort not only with current treatment but also with future treatment. As most dental visits are scheduled within a 6 to 12 month range, these patients may benefit from daily to weekly practice and more frequent community professional visits. Once the skills are generalized and maintained, the frequency of practice and visitation may be altered.

With all the techniques discussed, it is very important to communicate with parents before initiating any treatment in a developmentally challenged patient. The discussion should elicit expectations of the parent and the clinician and both should understand that visits may be long and that multiple visits may be required to accomplish the desired treatment.

CHALLENGES FOR THE OMS

Being one of the few surgical specialties in which procedures are performed quickly and on an outpatient basis, oral surgical treatment of the

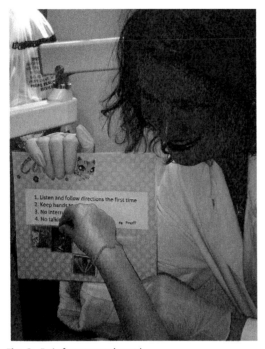

Fig. 2. Reinforcement board.

uncooperative pediatric patient is extremely challenging. Given the pace of ambulatory practice, there may be a need for the OMS to adopt unfamiliar concepts and techniques when faced with

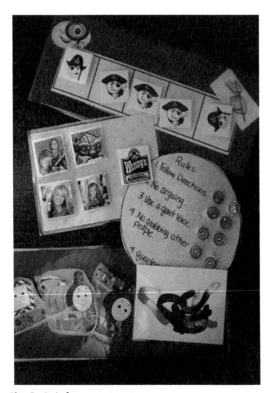

Fig. 3. Reinforcement systems.

children who exhibit behavioral challenges. Because of possibly significant drug interactions, potentially challenging anesthetic administration and recovery, and basic neurophysiologic differences in this subpopulation, a shift to nonpharmacologic management is desirable.

Adding to these challenges, it should be noted that in some children with behavioral issues, there are concomitant impairments of fine and gross motor coordination, which may have an effect on oral heath and treatment needs. These impairments may be caused by neurophysiologic issues associated with an underlying process, with effects extending beyond behavior. Motor incoordination may result in inadequate oral hygiene and an increased risk for dental treatment needs, including extractions. Highly sensory aversive individuals may avoid oral tasks, including tooth brushing, because of physical or auditory negative stimulation, and parents may lack an adequate understanding of the long-term sequelae of avoidance behavior. Practitioners should be encouraged to discuss such issues with parents and other professionals, including therapists and school personnel, to decrease the risk of oral health decline.

The OMS is well trained in pharmacology and very comfortable with anesthesia but generally has limited knowledge and training in the management of behavioral disorders. As such, many oral and maxillofacial surgery practitioners elect to treat most behaviorally challenged patients with pharmacologic means, including outpatient conscious sedation and general anesthesia. Complicating matters, the increased use of prescribed psychotropic drugs in this patient population may lead to significant interactions with the sedative-hypnotic agents typically used in the OMS's setting. Selective serotonin reuptake inhibitors, central adrenergic agonists, antipsychotics, benzodiazepines, tricyclic antidepressants, lithium, valproate, and carbamazepine have all been prescribed to treat the behavioral and psychological effects of disorders affecting mood, emotion, and behavior.[6] At present, the only drug approved by the Food and Drug Administration to treat symptoms of autism is risperidone (Risperdal). However, many medications are being tried on an off-label basis to control psychotic, obsessive-compulsive, and anxiety behaviors in children with mental illness, including autism.

With the increasing use of prescription drug management, side effects and complications must be anticipated and managed in an effort to ensure patient safety and produce successful treatment outcomes. It is critical that the surgeon is aware of potential drug interactions between medications prescribed by physicians treating patients and the pharmacologic agents used in oral and maxillofacial surgery. New medications are constantly being introduced into the market. One example is guanfacine (intuniv), an alpha A2 receptor antagonist manufactured in 2009, which may be prescribed. Current accurate documentation of medications is critical. Surgeons must educate themselves about all medications listed in the patient health history, updating the history and their knowledge with the introduction of new drugs. For example, in multiple controlled studies, naltrexone has been shown to decrease the aggressive behaviors in some patients with autism.[7–9] Consider the consequence of using an opioid medication as part of a sedative protocol in a patient using naltrexone, an opioid antagonist, for behavior control.

Supplemental therapies, vitamins, and diets are commonly used in this population. Parents may not be forthcoming with this information because of the stigma of alternative therapies and the misconception that these substances are less likely than standard pharmaceuticals to produce adverse drug reactions and interactions.

Additional consideration must be given to the communication and social difficulties associated with children with developmental delays and psychiatric illness. Classical autism, pervasive developmental disorder, and Asperger syndrome all contain aspects of language delay that may be both receptive and expressive. As such, children on this spectrum may not be able to understand simple commands and may also have difficulty processing and following commands. Simple one-step directions for treatment are most appropriate in this population. In the absence of a school- or home-based program for skill acquisition, video modeling, or social story formulation, the professional should be able to recommend or implement such procedures for the child.

CONSCIOUS SEDATION/GENERAL ANESTHESIA CONCERNS

Pediatric outpatient sedation and anesthesia have been performed safely in the ambulatory oral surgical setting with great success. Advances in monitoring and the availability of multiple medications, including reversal agents, have led to the safe administration of sedation in outpatient pediatric surgical environments. However, challenges are still faced, and the uncooperative child remains among the most challenging of the patients in the OMS's practice.

With uncooperative children, especially those with diagnosed mental illness and developmental delays, there are many factors that must be considered before finalizing a treatment protocol. Although most children can be managed with behavioral techniques and the use of nitrous oxide when indicated, a subset of this population still require sedation or general anesthesia to accomplish necessary oral surgical procedures. Pediatric patients with mental illness have a higher-than-normal anxiety level than neurotypical peers. These patients may also be challenged by the ability to maintain themselves in the chair for extended periods. They may become aggressive or combative during the visit and may have disabling sensory integration issues such that they have no ability to tolerate any procedures, including wearing a nitrous oxide nasal hood. Children with ASDs, in particular, react poorly to changes in routine, and this reaction can affect all aspects of the oral surgical visit. These children can often be identified before any treatment appointments by discussion with the referring clinician or family members. For children and adolescents, such as those described earlier, pharmacologic assistance may be required and sedation or general anesthesia should be considered.

All patients reporting for sedation and general anesthesia are expected to adhere to nothing-by-mouth instructions developed by the American Society of Anesthesiologists, which may make early morning appointments more attractive for many patients and highly desirable for the child with behavioral issuers. These children may have dysfunctional eating habits, diets, routines, and preferences, which make maintenance of the nothing-by-mouth status extremely difficult. Discussion should take place with the parent about dietary restrictions should any oral premedications with fluids be required. Children on the autism spectrum and with ADD/ADHD may be following restrictive diets, and parental information about these diets is critical. Dietary issues may also complicate electrolyte balance, and the results of recent laboratory testing should be obtained for children with significant dietary restrictions. Discussion with the child's pediatrician and/or nutritionist may help to avoid complications associated with fluid management and may permit collaboration in providing some perioperative dietary flexibility. Oral dosing of midazolam and diazepam has been effective in children with mild disorders, whereas oral ketamine is the most efficacious in moderate to severely combative patients.[10,11] Ketamine can be mixed with favored clear liquids provided these liquids do not violate the nothing-by-mouth recommendations in volume or consistency.

For children and adolescents who are moderately to severely combative and adhere to nothing by mouth, the intramuscular route of medication administration is most effective. Once adequately sedated, the choice to introduce an intravenous (IV) line and IV medications may be considered for ongoing titration to maintain appropriate levels of sedation and anesthesia. This intravenous introduction also ensures access for fluids, emergency medications, and reversal agents should they be required.

Through multiple studies, conscious sedation and general anesthesia have been shown to be safe in the population with autism. Medications such as midazolam, diazepam, propofol, ketamine, pentobarbital, and fentanyl have demonstrated efficacy in this group.[10–13] However, it should be noted that in one study, on a per-kilogram basis, the study group consisting of children with an ASD from ages 18 to 36 months has a significantly lower fentanyl requirement than the secondary group of children without autistic behaviors.[12] The same study elucidated that children with ASDs have no higher dose requirements than the general population for noninvasive imaging studies. Considering that oral surgical procedures are invasive by nature, the ability to correlate this data is questionable. However, consideration should be given to reducing the opioid dose in this group.

Also of note is a study that compared oral diazepam and midazolam for the sedation of patients with autism during dental treatment. The study concluded that midazolam was more effective than diazepam during portions of the procedure that were associated with increased stimulation.[10] The study also showed that although both diazepam and midazolam were effective, safe, and successfully used, midazolam was significantly more effective in managing the crying and movement often seen early in procedures.

Generally, outpatient sedation and general anesthesia are considered safe in this population. However, it is reasonable to consider hospital-based treatment in children and adolescents who are severely affected by mental illness and require complex and/or lengthy procedures. This decision must be made with the input of parents, therapists, pediatricians, anesthesiologists, and the oral health care provider. The ultimate goal is to restore oral health in the safest and most efficacious manner.

SUMMARY

Managing the uncooperative pediatric patient is a challenge for all health care providers. With the dramatic increase in the diagnosis of these disorders, all OMSs are faced with the behavioral, anesthetic, and surgical management of this patient population. The keys to successful management require an education about these disabilities, their associated features, the successful techniques available, and knowledge of alternate therapies. With these tools, the OMS can formulate and implement an individualized treatment plan based on all of the information gathered about each patient. With advancing knowledge and training in these areas, children and adolescents with mental illness and uncooperative behavior are managed successfully in the outpatient oral surgical practice.

REFERENCES

1. Satcher D. Goals. In: Reports of the surgeon general's, conference on children's mental health: a national action agenda. Washington, DC: Department of Health and Human Services; 2000. p. 1–5.
2. Satcher D. Conference summary-background. In: Reports of the surgeon general's conference on children's mental health: a national action agenda. Washington, DC: Department of Health and Human Services; 2000. p. 1–2.
3. Rice C. Prevalence of autism spectrum disorders—Autism and Developmental Disabilities Monitoring Network, United States, 2006. MMWR Surveill Summ; Atlanta (GA): 2009;58(SS10):1–20.
4. Barbaresi W, Katusic S, Colligan R, et al. How common is attention-deficit/hyperactivity disorder? Towards resolution of the controversy: results from a population-based study. Acta Paediatr Suppl 2007;93(s445):55–9.
5. Bellini S, Akullian J. A meta-analysis of video modeling and video self-modeling interventions for children and adolescents with autism spectrum disorders. Except Child 2007;73(3):264–87.
6. Weisz JR, Jensen PS. Efficacy and effectiveness of child and adolescent psychotherapy and pharmacotherapy. Ment Health Serv Res 1999;1(3):125–57.
7. Leboyer M, Bouvard MP, Launay JM, et al. Opiate hypothesis in infantile autism? Therapeutic trials with naltrexone. Encephale 1993;19(2):95–102.
8. Elchaar GM, Maisch NM, Augusto LM, et al. Efficacy and safety of naltrexone use in pediatric patients with autistic disorder. Ann Pharmacother 2006;40(6):1086–95.
9. Rossignol DA. Novel and emerging treatments for autism spectrum disorders: a systematic review. Ann Clin Psychiatry 2009;21(4):213–36.

10. Pisalchaiyong T, Trairatvorakul C, Jirakijja J, et al. Comparison of the effectiveness of oral diazepam and midazolam for the sedation of autistic patients during dental treatment. Pediatr Dent 2005;27(3):198–206.

11. Van Der Walt J, Moran C. An audit of perioperative management of autistic children. Paediatr Anaesth 2001;11(4):401–8.

12. Ross AK, Hazlett HC, Garrett N, et al. Moderate sedation for MRI in young children with autism. Pediatr Radiol 2005;35(9):867–71.

13. Tsang RW, Solow HL, Ananthanarayan C, et al. Daily general anaesthesia for radiotherapy in uncooperative patients: ingredients for successful management. Clin Oncol 2001;13(6):416–21.

Discussing Adverse Outcomes with Patients and Families

Rachel Bluebond-Langner, MD[a],
Eduardo D. Rodriguez, MD, DDS[b],
Albert W. Wu, MD, MPH[c],*

KEYWORDS
- Disclosure • Adverse event • Near miss • Apology

CASE 1

A 23-year-old man with an unremarkable medical history requires the surgical extraction of maxillary and mandibular third molars. The patient reports a strong gag reflex and prefers surgical extraction with intravenous (IV) sedation. The oral surgeon is accredited and well qualified to administer anesthesia. After IV sedation with propofol, midazolam, and fentanyl, maxillary and mandibular nerve blocks are performed without difficulty, except for an occasional gag response. After allowing appropriate time for anesthesia, the surgeon proceeds to place a throat pack but is unable to do so because of the strong gag response. The surgeon administers additional propofol to overcome the gag. The patient becomes hypoxic, and the surgeon responds appropriately by ventilating the patient with an Ambu-mask until the O_2 saturation reaches 100%. The surgeon proceeds to surgically remove the mandibular third molars uneventfully, and chromic gut sutures are placed without difficulty. The first maxillary third molar is removed without difficulty. However, after luxation, the remaining maxillary third molar with convergent roots quickly rolls out of the socket into the pharynx. Without a throat pack, the surgeon attempts to retract the tooth with the Yankauer suction tip but proceeds to push it deeper into the hypopharynx. After some struggle the tooth is irretrievable. A chest radiograph reveals that the maxillary third molar is located in the right main bronchus. The patient is admitted to the hospital, undergoes bronchoscopic extraction of the third molar, and is discharged the following morning.

CASE 2

A 19-year-old woman requests surgical extraction of affected mandibular third molars with IV sedation. The surgeon is accredited and well qualified to administer anesthesia. After IV sedation with propofol, midazolam, and fentanyl, maxillary and mandibular nerve blocks are performed without difficulty. After allowing appropriate time for anesthesia, the oral surgeon proceeds to place a throat pack without difficulty. The surgical assistant informs the surgeon that the surgical handpiece does not have a protective guard and that the surgeon needs to wait for 30 minutes for the next available handpiece. The surgeon decides to proceed because there are several other patients scheduled. The right mandibular third molar is deeply affected with divergent roots. Despite an unfavorable split of the tooth, the surgeon

[a] Division of Plastic and Reconstructive Surgery, Johns Hopkins School of Medicine, 8th Floor, 600 North Caroline Street, Baltimore, MD 21287, USA
[b] Division of Plastic and Reconstructive Surgery, R Adams Cowley Shock Trauma Center, and the University of Maryland Medical Systems, 22 South Greene Street, Baltimore, MD 21201, USA
[c] Department of Health Policy and Management, Johns Hopkins Bloomberg School of Public Health, 624 North Broadway Street, Room 653, Baltimore, MD 21205, USA
* Corresponding author.
E-mail address: awu@jhsph.edu

Oral Maxillofacial Surg Clin N Am 22 (2010) 471–479
doi:10.1016/j.coms.2010.07.004

struggles to remove the crown and embedded root tips. The surgeon soon recognizes that the unprotected burr shank has caused a severe third-degree burn involving the entire upper and lower lip commissure, which is surgically uncorrectable. The surgeon places gauze in the tooth sockets and applies antibiotic ointment to the commissure. At the 3-month follow-up the patient does not complain of paresthesias or pain. However, she is concerned with the hypertrophic scarring and hypopigmentation of the lip commissure.

ERRORS AND ORAL SURGERY

Complications and undesired outcomes happen to some patients of virtually all physicians, at all stages in their careers. Bad outcomes can be a consequence of disease processes, the premorbid condition of the patient, or the errors that occur in the process of health care. These errors include, but are by no means confined to, surgeon error. Regardless of the reason for the bad outcome, the surgeon is obligated to discuss the event with the patient and the family. Disclosing and discussing these events and outcomes with the patients is challenging and often painful for both the patient and the physician. Worries about the potential legal consequences of the incident, and that disclosure might trigger a lawsuit, make the process still more difficult.

Human beings always make errors. A medical error has been defined "as the failure of a planned action to be completed as intended (ie, error of execution) or the use of a wrong plan to achieve an aim (ie, error of planning)."[1] An adverse event is an injury caused by medical care. Identifying some event as an adverse one does not imply error, negligence, or poor quality of care. Rather, such identification indicates an undesired outcome that results from diagnosis or treatment as opposed to the underlying disease process.

Error, bad outcome, negligence, and lawsuits are distinct entities that are often confused, particularly in the minds of physicians involved in adverse events. In fact, not all errors are negligent, and lawsuits may occur in the setting of a bad outcome despite the absence of any error. Some errors result in patient harm, whereas others do not (**Fig. 1**). Grading schemes are available to quantify the extent of harm, which may range from none to death and which may involve physical and other kinds of injury (**Table 1**). Errors that do not cause patient harm either because they do not reach the patient or because they reach the patient but cause no harm are referred to as "near misses" or "close calls." Near misses

are sometimes due to chance, sometimes to patient resilience, and sometimes to actions taken to prevent or mitigate harm.

Bad outcomes and errors that result in patient harm should be discussed with the patient, both because there is an ethical obligation to do so and because patients expect and want this to be done. There is less of an imperative to disclose a near miss, but disclosure can still be beneficial; in addition, there is little risk of litigation.

ORAL SURGERY AND DISCLOSURE

There are some factors related to the practice of oral surgery that make the difficult process of disclosure a little easier. Because most procedures in oral surgery are done on an elective basis, an established patient-doctor relationship exists before the procedure or surgery. The potential risks and adverse outcomes of the operation have been discussed, often at length, and the patient, in giving consent, should have had at least some understanding of complications that could result from the surgery. However, what is included in a consent discussion and the signed consent form is not necessarily actually heard or understood. Even if a potential complication is mentioned during the consent process, it does not necessarily make it easier to accept an adverse outcome. Therefore it behooves the oral surgeon to take advantage of the opportunity to establish a rapport with the patient and build trust. An office visit prior to the procedure in which questions are answered and the patient is provided with literature and the consent document to take home and review can help to prepare the patient for the potential of a negative outcome.

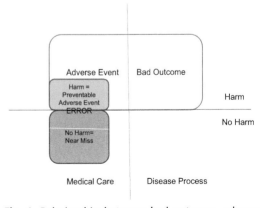

Fig. 1. Relationship between bad outcome, adverse event, error, negligence, and lawsuit.

Table 1
UHC definition of different types of medical incidents

Near miss	Unsafe conditions
	The event did not reach the individual because of chance alone
	The event did not reach the individual because of active recovery by caregivers
Event caused no harm	The event reached the individual but did not cause harm (an error of omission, such as a missed medication dose, does reach the patient)
	The event reached the individual, and additional monitoring was required to prevent harm
Event caused harm	The individual experienced temporary harm and required treatment or intervention
	The individual experienced temporary harm and required initial or prolonged hospitalization
	The individual experienced permanent harm
	The individual experienced harm and required intervention necessary to sustain life
Death	The individual died

Abbreviation: UHC, University HealthSystem Consortium.

On the other hand, there are also aspects of oral surgical procedures that might make it more difficult to disclose an adverse outcome. A portion of patients requiring oral surgery present for completely elective procedures and do not anticipate complications. Because of these expectations, the tolerance for a complication or a less than perfect result is likely to be reduced. In these cases, it is of utmost importance to emphasize preoperatively and repeatedly that there are serious and real risks associated with any procedure. Showing photographs of excellent as well as poor outcomes and even complications can help to prepare the patient for possible adverse outcomes.

THE ETHICAL DUTY TO DISCLOSE

There is an ethical obligation for physicians and health care organizations to disclose adverse events to patients and/or their families. The ethical obligations to disclose an adverse event are based on fiduciary responsibility, the principles of autonomy, truth telling, and respect for patients, and professional standards. The role of the fiduciary can be traced back to the Roman law. The responsibilities of a fiduciary come into play when a party is entrusted with the management and responsibility of another's property. Now, the fiduciary has the responsibility to make decisions regarding the property, which would solely benefit the first party. Similarly, when patients entrust their care into the hands of physicians, the physicians become the patients' fiduciaries. Physicians are then required to act in the best interests of their patients.[2]

A crucial aspect of acting in patients' best interest is enabling them to make autonomous decisions about their care. To make an autonomous decision, a patient must be fully informed about his or her condition and potential consequences of various courses of action.[3,4] After an adverse event, the patient must be given the facts related to the incident to allow decision making regarding future care. Thus, disclosure gives the patient the opportunity to understand recommendations and to proceed with care, whether it is provided by the current physician or another physician. Disclosure also allows the patient the option of seeking compensation. If the patient is not made aware of what happened in the case of a preventable adverse event, he or she may be deprived of the needed compensation.

The physician's obligation to tell the truth is a core value in medical ethics.[3–5] The duty of truth telling is consistent with the principle of respect for patients. Truth telling is closely linked to the ability of the patient to make autonomous decisions and seek remediation, and to the physician who fills the role as the patient's fiduciary.

Professional standards dictate open disclosure of adverse events. The American Medical Association Ethics Manual reads, "physicians should disclose to patients information about procedural or judgment errors made in the course of care if such information is material to the patient's well-being. Errors do not necessarily constitute improper, negligent, or unethical behavior, but failure to disclose them may."[6,7]

The Joint Commission[8] states that, "[p]atients and when appropriate, their families, are informed about the outcomes of care, including unanticipated outcomes." These and other professional standards have led organizations to develop their own policies for handling medical errors. For example, the Johns Hopkins Hospital's Medical Error Disclosure Policy, developed in 2001, states, "[i]t is the right of the patient to receive information about clinically relevant medical errors. The JHH has an obligation to disclose information regarding these errors to the patient in a prompt, clear and honest manner."[9] These policies are readily adopted by health care organizations because they are entirely consistent with the core mission of the institutions.

BENEFITS OF DISCLOSURE

In addition to the ethical arguments and the benefits to the individual patients, developing an open disclosure policy can help an organization promote patient safety. Acknowledging the occurrence of error and patient harm is necessary to set expectations about open disclosure and encourage subsequent dialogue regarding the error. Disclosure helps to normalize error, decrease the associated stigma around error, and establish a culture that promotes safety. Making a public commitment to being open about medical errors can accelerate this process and may also help to calibrate patient expectations about the potential for adverse outcomes.

BARRIERS TO DISCLOSURE

Despite the ethical duty to disclose and the consensus that disclosing an adverse event is in the best interests of the patient, the surgeon, and the medical profession, many adverse events are not disclosed. Even when disclosure occurs, it may be incomplete or misleading. Omission of pertinent facts may be unintentional or may be done in an attempt to protect the surgeon and the medical staff.[10] Regardless of the intention, inaccurate or partial disclosure does not allow the patient to make an informed decision, erodes the patient-doctor relationship, and creates distrust.

Adverse events are distressing for both physicians and patients.[11] Physicians respond to making a mistake with shock, fear, remorse, guilt, anger, and self-doubt. The physician may feel profoundly isolated and may not know where to turn for help or advice.[12] The prospect of disclosing an adverse event and the resulting emotional reaction from a patient and the family is also upsetting and may discourage disclosure.

In general, it is difficult to admit failure of any kind, which is particularly true in medicine in which

the promise of advances in practice and technology and the stories of miraculous recoveries contribute to a shared expectation of perfection by patients and health providers.[13] In this context, errors are viewed as a deviant rather than an inevitable part of medical practice, and are stigmatized by both the public and peers. Both disclosure and reporting of incidents are then driven underground. Reason[14] describes a "vulnerable system syndrome" in which managers further reinforce this vicious circle by castigating individuals associated with the rare incident that comes to light. This syndrome assures that further disclosures will be uncommon.

LEGAL IMPLICATIONS OF DISCLOSURE

Fear of legal ramifications is another important barrier to disclosure and can impair one's ability to divulge the full truth. The idea that "anything you say can be used against you" is prevalent. Many physicians believe that full disclosure is tantamount to an admission of guilt and increases the chances of being sued.[12,15] Ironically, research and anecdotes suggest the opposite. Many patients believe that doctors withhold information,[16] and if anything, when patients are told about what happened in a candid, clear, and honest manner, they are less likely to sue.[15,17] One Internet survey found that full disclosure strengthened the doctor-patient relationship and could reduce the desire to sue.[18] A comparison of different methods of disclosure found that full disclosure resulted in greater trust and satisfaction and no increased likelihood of seeking legal advice.[19] Other studies have found that patients were more likely to trust physicians who played an active role in disclosing a serious error,[20] whereas inadequate disclosure may increase the likelihood of seeking legal advice[19] or filing a malpractice claim.[21]

On the other hand, full disclosure may make those who are aware of an injury less likely to sue. Studdert and colleagues[22] have suggested that lawsuits may result if patients are made aware that they were injured by a previously unsuspected error. A simple lack of information about what happened combined with a bad outcome can lead to a patient's decision to sue. Nevertheless, Vincent and colleagues[23] have found that patients or family members take legal action not only because of the original adverse event but also because of the lack of information and poor handling of the incident.

The experience of the Veterans Affairs (VA) Medical Center in Lexington, Kentucky is instructive. Since 1987, the Kentucky VA Medical Center has had an adverse event policy that emphasizes the duty of the physician to notify the patient (or family) if there was an error in their care. The number of liability claims was moderate, and the total payouts of the Medical Center were lower than those of comparable institutions. Also, out of 88 claims filed in a 7-year period, only 8 proceeded to the federal court where 7 were dismissed, and the one that proceeded to trial was found in favor of the VA Medical Center.[24]

The University of Michigan Medical Center modeled their program for handling adverse events on the Lexington VA Medical Center program. The University of Michigan Medical Center's program, begun in 2003, has met with notable and demonstrable success.[25] The center reports a reduction in claims and lawsuits from 265 in 2002 to 120 in 2005 to the current 10-year low. Average litigation and attorney fees have decreased from $65,000 to $30,000 per case. Time to completion of cases has also been reduced from 1160 to 300 days on average. Perhaps most compelling is the ability of this program to reduce the Medical Center's indemnity reserves (held to cover the possibility of anticipated payments) from $72 million to $20 million.

HOW TO DISCLOSE

Perhaps the most easily remedied barrier to disclosure is the lack of instruction in communication: physicians are not trained on how to disclose a medical error and as a result have a harder time fulfilling their duty to disclose. Although disclosure is something that all physicians will be faced with, there is little opportunity for formal training.

What should be said in explaining an adverse event? Although disclosure should never be scripted, there are a few general principles to follow. The initial statement is important because the phenomenon of emotional flooding may result in that statement being the only one that the patient remembers. Therefore, as in the case of breaking bad news, the disclosure of a medical error could begin with a statement such as "I am afraid I have bad news." An initial disclosure discussion should include an explanation of what occurred, what will happen next, an apology, and an acknowledgment of responsibility. It is vital not to make assumptions about what the patient knows. Before discussing details of the adverse event, the patient should be asked about what they already know. By determining the extent of the patient's knowledge, the physician can calibrate the discussion to the patient's level of information and understanding.

Apology is a key element of the discussion; patients expect it. Patients have both informational and emotional needs in these discussions. It is important to convey empathy and regret, which can be done through words, tone of voice, as well as demeanor and posture. At all points during the discussion, the patient should be given the opportunity to react, express emotions, and ask questions. Care should be taken to be responsive to the patient's cues and tempo rather than responding to every comment immediately, rushing the conversation, cutting the patient off, or talking over the patient. It is important to pause frequently to provide the patient with the opportunity to absorb the information, ask questions, and make comments. Important facts may have to be repeated more than once. Questions should be asked to ascertain whether or not the patient understands what is being said.

It is also important to explain expected future consequences and what can be done to prevent similar events from happening again. A complication presents a new and threatening problem and can leave the patient with a fear of abandonment. It is important to convey to the patient that the surgeon continues to be committed to the treatment and resolution of the complication even if additional specialists become involved. Reaching out to specialists is not a sign of weakness and often can be a source of support to the surgeon and the patient.

It is likely that patients will be upset to learn about the error, and they may react with anger toward the physician. Such a reaction should be expected; it is unrealistic to expect that the patient will accept the news with equanimity, and physicians should take great care to manage their own reactions in response to those of the patients. The physician should work to avoid being defensive or angry when confronted with questions from the patient or family member.

THE DISCLOSURE PROCESS

It is important is to view the disclosure of an adverse event as a part of ongoing dialogue between patient and physician about the patient's condition, decision making, and what is occurring in the patient's health care.

It can be helpful to think about the disclosure process as a special case of breaking bad news because this is something that is more familiar to all physicians.[26] Once an adverse outcome has been recognized or the effects of the error are noticed, immediate steps should be taken to prevent, rectify, or minimize the harm caused by the error (**Fig. 2**). The patient and/or the family should be notified as soon as possible after the adverse event has been identified. An investigation

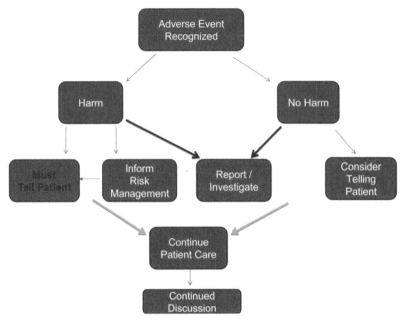

Fig. 2. Disclosure process.

should be initiated into the cause of the adverse event, and strategies should be deployed to reduce the probability of recurrence. Communication regarding the incident does not absolutely end with the initial disclosure discussion. Just as patient care continues, communication with the patient should continue as more is learned from investigation of the incident and as changes to the patient's care are made. If significant changes are made at the organizational level to improve safety, the patient should be notified about this as well.

In cases in which the patient is not harmed (a near miss or close call), disclosure of the incident is discretionary. Virtually no health care organization mandates disclosure of near-miss events. However, the incident should still be reported to the organization or reporting system so that an investigation into the cause of the error can be launched. Near-miss events are more frequent than adverse ones and generally stem from the same causes. Therefore such events can be used to identify important system flaws that have the potential to cause future errors and injury. Studying near-miss events can also identify valuable strategies that allowed recovery from incidents that otherwise might have caused harm. In addition, health care workers are likely to be less inhibited about discussing the incidents freely because there is much less worry about disciplinary consequences. Near misses should be looked on as opportunities to improve patient safety.[27]

Although the disclosure of a near miss is discretionary, it is also important to keep in mind what the patients want. Multiple studies have indicated that patients wish to be notified of virtually all errors in their care, not just those that cause harm.[17,28] Being open with a patient regarding all errors (both those resulting in and not resulting in adverse events) can help to build the patient's trust and enable the patient full autonomy regarding medical decisions. The primary constraint may be that discussion of all errors is not always practical. In some settings, disclosing all errors that occur in a patient's care would burden both caregivers and patients. A compromise is represented by the VA Medical Center's policy, which encourages disclosing all events that require a change in plan or writing a note about the incident.[29]

WHEN AN ADVERSE EVENT SHOULD BE DISCLOSED

An adverse event should be disclosed as soon as it is recognized, which may be in the initial postprocedure discussion with the patient or the family, or in some cases during a follow-up visit. Discussion with risk management representatives or seeking legal advice prior to disclosure can help guide and support the physician. When there is a serious adverse event, this discussion is mandatory to help optimize outcomes for all parties concerned. If the adverse event is identified after the patient has left the office, the patient should be asked to return for a discussion in person, if possible, rather than discussing it over the phone. This act reinforces trusts and communicates a sense of commitment.

WHO SHOULD DISCLOSE THE ADVERSE EVENT

The physician who is ultimately responsible for the patient and procedure (usually the attending surgeon) should generally disclose the error or event. Patients usually want "their doctor" to have these discussions with them. However, it may be helpful for other health professionals, such as nurses, to participate, if they can help to explain what happened in the incident. There are arguments for allowing the initial discussion to be entirely clinical in focus, concentrating on informing the patient about his or her health and course of treatment. A risk management representative may be helpful but his or her presence may also make the patient wary—it may be best to save this meeting for a later discussion, should this be needed.

WHAT SHOULD BE DISCLOSED

Deciding what to disclose to a patient and the family can be difficult. If a situation requires a note, an additional procedure, or a change in the stated plan, the physician should disclose the error to the patient. The initial disclosure should include a statement of the anticipated initial plan and then what actually happened. If there are parts of the story that are not yet known, the surgeon should state them. It is important to avoid speculation; there have been many incidents in which remorseful physicians have disclosed things that they did not do, complicating later discussions when these statements had to be retracted. The patient should be reassured that as more information is obtained it will be shared. Full disclosure leads to greater trust. Patients appreciate prompt disclosure, honesty, and the opportunity for ongoing dialogue.

WHAT TO SAY, AND HOW TO DISCLOSE

Disclosure is difficult, and every disclosure discussion is in some ways unique. No single guideline or checklist can provide all the guidance that a physician may need when disclosing an error. However, there are some basic strategies to keep in mind when conducting these discussions. The discussion should occur in a private and quiet location. Discussions can be stressful and upsetting for both patients and their families and health care workers, and providing privacy respects this stressful situation.

It is important to try to make the patients feel as comfortable as possible when they are likely to feel vulnerable and powerless. It is helpful for the physician to begin by making eye contact with the patient and put oneself on the same level.[26] If the patient is sitting the physician should sit. If the patient opts to remain standing, the physician should do the same. Placing physical barriers, such as a desk or hospital bed, between the physician and patient during disclosure should be avoided.

The initial statement is important because the phenomenon of emotional flooding may result in it being the only thing that the patient remembers. Therefore, as in the case of breaking bad news, the disclosure of a medical error could begin with a statement such as "I am afraid I have bad news." It is vital not to make assumptions about what the patient knows. Before discussing details of the adverse event, the patient should be asked what they already know. By determining the extent of the patient's knowledge, the physician can calibrate the discussion to the patient's level of information and understanding.

Physicians should not rush, but should pause frequently to provide the patient with the opportunity to absorb the information, ask questions, and make comments. Important facts may have to be repeated more than once. Questions should be asked to ascertain whether or not the patient understands what is being said.

It is likely that the patients will be upset to learn about the error and may react with anger toward the physician. This reaction should be expected; it is unrealistic to expect that patients will accept the news with equanimity, and physicians should take great care to manage their reactions in response to those of the patients. The physician should work to avoid being defensive or angry when confronted with questions from the patient or family member.

The discussion should include an explanation of what happened, a sincere apology, and assurance that an investigation will be conducted. Strong emotional reactions should be handled by validating them and empathizing with the patient. Keeping this in mind will help the patient feel more respected, heard, and comforted.

APOLOGY

In repeated studies, patients have emphasized 3 things that they expect to hear in a disclosure: a description of what happened, assurance that the problem will be investigated and fixed, and an apology.[17,18,30] It is crucial to apologize for an adverse event. An apology is what patients expect and want, and they may cope better if they understand that the physician also feels badly about an incident. A full disclosure including a sincere apology conveys respect for the patient and also allows the potential of forgiveness. However, the physician should keep in mind that although disclosure and apology are necessary for forgiveness to occur, they do not guarantee that the patient will forgive the physician. Forgiveness may take a long time or may never occur. However, without an apology there is no basis to allow the process of forgiveness to begin.[31]

Physicians should strive to empathize with what the patient experiences in the discussion. Empathy includes validating the patient's emotions, conveying a sense of understanding the link to one's own actions, and offering support. Listening to the patient helps to communicate respect.[26] It is also helpful to express one's own emotions, for example, "I feel terrible that this has happened," with the recognition that the discussion is primarily focused on the patient rather than the doctor.

The apology should be sincere and appropriate to what is known about the incident. Patients want someone to take responsibility for what happened.[18,30] In the case of individual responsibility, the physician should say, "I am sorry that I did this." However, situations are often complex, involving multiple system factors, and the error may not be any one individual's responsibility. In cases such as this, the physician can still accept responsibility on behalf of the health care team or institution saying, "I am sorry that this happened, we are responsible for this." The importance of accepting responsibility is great, but it also crucial not to blame other individuals during the disclosure. "Jousting" should always be avoided; when making the disclosure, the physician should take care not to name, blame, or criticize others involved in the incident.

Apologizing is not the same as admitting guilt. There are no data to suggest that apologizing increases the chance of litigation. Anecdotal evidence suggests that apology sometimes averted a claim.[32] Anecdotal evidence also suggests that when an apology is made in mediations, the apology assists in resolving the case. More than 20 US states have now passed legislation that make an apology inadmissible in a court of law.[33]

SUMMARY

Bad outcomes and errors occur to every surgeon at some point in his or her career. It is important to acknowledge these events and discuss them honestly with the patient. When approaching the discussion, apology, acceptance of responsibility, and commitment to continuing to care closely for the patient after the event are key to preserving a working patient-doctor relationship. After disclosure of the medical error, it is important to be proactive in maintaining contact with the patient. Involving risk management early can be a source of support and guidance for the physician.

REFERENCES

1. Institute of Medicine. To err is human: building a safer health system. Washington, DC: National Academy Press; 2000.
2. Perkins HS. The physician as fiduciary: the basis for an ethics of patient care. In: Stein JH, editor. In: Internal medicine, vol. 2. Boston: Little, Brown & Co; 1990. p. 2448–50.
3. Vogel J, Delgado R. To tell the truth: physicians' duty to disclose medical mistakes. UCLA Law Rev 1980; 28(52):52–94.
4. Wu AW, Cavanaugh TA, McPhee SJ, et al. To tell the truth: ethical and practical issues in disclosing medical mistakes to patients. J Gen Intern Med 1997;12:770–5.
5. Gallagher SM. Truth telling. Ostomy Wound Manage 1998;44(11):17–9.
6. Ethics manual. Fourth edition. American College of Physicians. Ann Intern Med 1998;128:576–94.
7. AMA Council on Ethical and Judicial Affairs. Code of medical ethics: current opinions with annotations. Chicago: AMA; 1997. sect 8.12:125.
8. Joint Commission on the Accreditation of Healthcare Organizations. RI.1.1.2. July 1, 2001.
9. Johns Hopkins Hospital. Error disclosure policy. Interdisciplinary clinical practice manual. Available at: www.insidehopkinsmedicine.org/icpm. Accessed July 17, 2010.
10. Chan DK, Gallagher TH, Reznick R, et al. How surgeons disclose medical errors to patients: a study using standardized patients. Surgery 2005;138(5): 851–8.
11. Wu AW. Medical error: the second victim. The doctor who makes the mistake needs help too. Br Med J 2000;320:726–7.
12. Gallagher TH, Waterman AD, Ebers AG, et al. Patients and physicians' attitudes regarding the disclosure of medical errors. JAMA 2003;289(8): 1001–7.
13. Baylis F. Errors in medicine: nurturing truthfulness. J Clin Ethics 1997;8(4):336–40.
14. Reason JT. Human error. New York: Cambridge University Press; 1990.
15. Witman AB, Park DM, Hardin SB. How do patients want physicians to handle mistakes? A survey of

internal medicine patients in an academic setting. Arch Intern Med 1996;156:2565–9.

16. Itoh K, Andersen HB, Madsen MD, et al. Patient views of adverse events: comparisons of self-reported healthcare staff attitudes with disclosure of accident information. Appl Ergon 2006;37(4):513–23.

17. Mazor KM, Simon SR, Yood RA, et al. Health plan members' views about disclosure of medical errors. Ann Intern Med 2004;140(6):409–18, E419–23.

18. Schwappach DL, Koeck CM. What makes an error unacceptable? A factorial survey on the disclosure of medical errors. Int J Qual Health Care 2004;16(4): 317–26.

19. Mazor KM, Reed GW, Yood RA, et al. Disclosure of medical errors: what factors influence how patients respond? J Gen Intern Med 2006;21(7):704–10.

20. Fisseni G, Pentzek M, Abholz HH. Responding to serious medical error in general practice—consequences for the GPs involved: analysis of 75 cases from Germany. Fam Pract 2008;25(1):9–13.

21. Kachalia A, Shojania KG, Hofer TP, et al. Does full disclosure of medical errors affect malpractice liability? The jury is still out. Jt Comm J Qual Saf 2003;29(10):503–11.

22. Studdert DM, Mello MM, Gawande AA, et al. Disclosure of medical injury to patients: an improbable risk management strategy. Health Aff 2006;26(1):215–26.

23. Vincent C, Young M, Phillips A. Why do people sue doctors? A study of patients and relatives taking legal action. Lancet 1994;343(8913):609–13.

24. Kraman SS, Hamm G. Risk management: extreme honesty may be the best policy. Ann Intern Med 1999;131(12):963–7.

25. Boothman RC, Blackwell AC, Campbell DA, et al. A better approach to medical malpractice claims? The University of Michigan experience. J Health Life Sci Law 2009;2(2):125–59.

26. Buckman R. How to break bad news: a guide for health care professionals. Baltimore (MD): The Johns Hopkins University Press; 1992.

27. Wu AW. Is there an obligation to disclose near-misses in medical care? In: Sharpe VA, editor. Accountability: patient safety and policy reform. Washington, DC: Georgetown University Press; 2004. p. 135–42.

28. Hobgood C, Peck CR, Gilbert B, et al. Medical errors-what and when: what do patients want to know? Acad Emerg Med 2002;9:1156–61.

29. National Ethics Committee of the Veterans Health Administration. Disclosing adverse events to patients. Washington, DC: National Center for Ethics in Health Care, Veterans Health Administration, Department of Veteran Affairs; 2003.

30. Hingorani M, Wong T, Vafidis G. Patients' and doctors' attitudes to amount of information given after unintended injury during treatment: cross sectional, questionnaire survey. Br Med J 1999; 318:640–1.

31. Berlinger N. Avoiding cheap grace: medical harm, patient safety, and the culture(s) of forgiveness. Hastings Cent Rep 2003;33(6):28–36.

32. Zimmerman R. Doctors' new tool to fight lawsuits: saying 'I'm Sorry'. Wall Street Journal, May 18, 2005;A1.

33. Cohen JR. Toward candor after error: the first apology law. Harv Health Policy Rev 2004;5(1):21–4.

Understanding and Managing Patients with Chronic Pain

Richard P. Szumita, DDS[a,b,c,d,*],
Paul M. Szumita, PharmD, BCPS[e,f,g], Nancy Just, PhD, ABPP[h,i,j]

KEYWORDS
- Pain • Chronic pain • Cognitive behavioral therapy
- Analgesics

Dentistry has long been associated with the management of patients suffering from pain. Indeed, many of the advancements in early forms of anesthesia were discovered by and used by dentists in an effort to control the inevitable pain associated with dental procedures, predominantly dental extractions. Pain and anxiety control have remained a staple of dental education at the predoctoral and postdoctoral levels. Specifically, the specialty of oral and maxillofacial surgery has had at its core the foundations of anesthesia and pain and anxiety control. The specialty has continued to research and use various treatment strategies in the management of patients' pain. However, along with daily successes, every practitioner must remember that pain is diverse and complex. Research and treatment experience are expanding our knowledge of the mechanisms producing the experience of pain, and have revealed clinically significant differences between acute pain at one end of the pain spectrum and chronic pain at the other. Because most oral and maxillofacial surgeons manage acute pain and anxiety as part of the fabric of daily practice, clinicians must not bias diagnostic and management strategies in terms of acute pain paradigms. For chronic pain, as with all other conditions to be managed, a thorough understanding of pathophysiology is the foundation needed for effective management.

Previous editions of the *Oral and Maxillofacial Surgery Clinics of North America* have covered the diagnosis and management of chronic facial pain extensively. In fact, the *Clinics* were an important reference source used while researching for this article. The reader is well advised to refer to these reference sources to compile a complete database on this topic.[1–12] Rather than restating this material, the goal of this article is to refamiliarize the reader with clinical pearls helpful in the management of patients with chronic pain conditions. The authors also hope to highlight the

The authors have nothing to disclose.

[a] Oral and Maxillofacial Surgery Residency Training Program, St Joseph's Regional Medical Center, 703 Main Street Paterson, NJ 07503, USA

[b] Department of Dentistry, St Joseph's Regional Medical Center, 703 Main Street Paterson, NJ 07503, USA

[c] Department of Dentistry and Oral and Maxillofacial Surgery, School of Health and Medical Sciences, McQuaid Hall Seton Hall University, South Orange, NJ 07079, USA

[d] Private Practice, 30 West Century Road, Paramus, NJ 07652 and 55 East Main Street, Little Falls, NJ 07424, USA

[e] Department of Pharmacy Services, Brigham and Women's Hospital, Pharmacy Administration; L-2, 75 Francis Street, Boston, MA 02115, USA

[f] Critical Care, Northeastern University, 360 Huntington Avenue, Bouve College of Pharmacy and Health Sciences, 206 Mugar Building, Boston, MA, USA

[g] Critical Care, University of Rhode Island, College of Pharmacy, Fogarty Hall, 41 Lower College Road Kingston, RI 02881, USA

[h] American Academy of Clinical Psychology, PO Box 700341, San Antonio, TX 78270, USA

[i] American Board of Professional Psychology, 600 Market Street, Suite 300, Chapel Hill, NC 27516, USA

[j] Advanced Psychological Specialists, One Prospect Street, Suites 5–7, Ridgewood, NJ 07450, USA

* Corresponding author. 30 West Century Road, #210, Paramus, NJ 07652.
E-mail address: szumitar@sjhmc.org

Oral Maxillofacial Surg Clin N Am 22 (2010) 481–494
doi:10.1016/j.coms.2010.07.005

interplay of chronic pain and psychology as it relates to the oral and maxillofacial surgery patient. To that end, this article outlines and reviews the neurophysiology of pain, the definitions of pain, conditions encountered by the oral and maxillofacial surgeon that produce chronic pain, the psychological impact and comorbidities associated with patients experiencing chronic pain conditions, and concepts of multimodal treatment for patients experiencing chronic pain conditions.

PAIN THEORIES

Pain is a ubiquitous experience and a necessary function in human existence. Attempts to explain pain have been recorded throughout history and across many cultures. Early explanations were based on observations and superstitions. One of the first recorded theories that attempted to explain pain through scientific thought was the specificity theory.

Specificity Theory

In the 1600s, Descartes[13] proposed the specificity theory of pain. The theory postulated that a specific set of cutaneous receptors delivers signals from the periphery to the brain. When stimulated, these receptors—cold, warm, pain, and touch—signaled the brain with their specific messages. This theory presumed that receptors are differentiated and specialized and that there is a one-to-one relationship between the intensity of the particular stimulus and the experience of the particular sensation.

Pattern Theory

Another early theory, the pattern theory, proposed that receptors were undifferentiated, and that a specific pattern of stimulation was transmitted from the periphery directly to the brain. It was this "pattern" of stimulation that the brain would decipher as pain, pressure, cold, hot, and so forth. which explained the experience of pain.[13]

Gate Control Theory

Although commendable for their attempts to explain pain transmission scientifically, the specificity and pattern theories could not account for many conditions seen in clinical practice. In 1965, Melzack and Wall[13] proposed the gate control theory of pain, which proposes the existence of a "gating" mechanism between the sensory stimuli in the periphery and the processing of the stimuli within the central nervous system. The "gate" was thought to be in the substantia gelatinosa layer in the dorsal horn of the spinal cord,

where the various afferent (sensory) fibers terminate. This mechanism was thought to modulate nociceptive input entering the central nervous system. The theory proposes that nociceptive and non-nociceptive input from the periphery is transmitted to the substantia gelatinosa where the signals compete with each other. The non-nociceptive input activates interneuronal systems that inhibit transmission of the nociceptive signals to higher levels in the nervous system.

Additional modulation is then provided through downward signals from the central nervous system (CNS). The brain processes nociceptive input and influences further transmission by "signaling" down to the "gate." This process provides an opportunity for a patient to influence the pain response by altering these downward signals. In short, this is a neuroanatomical explanation for the "mind-body" connection. Although current pain theory differs somewhat from the ideas of Melzack and Wall, it is their work that established a strong foundation for our current understanding of how pain is perceived.

THE NEUROPHYSIOLOGY OF PAIN

Pain is initiated by the excitation of nociceptors, receptors that respond to noxious stimuli. Nociceptors are free nerve endings found in abundance in the skin, periosteum, arterial walls, joint surfaces, falx cerebri, and the tentorium cerebelli.[14] Deep structures are much more sparsely innervated. The impulses from the stimulation of these receptors are carried to the CNS in one of two ways: fast transmission of fast pain and slower transmission of slow pain. In fast pain, impulses are carried on larger diameter, myelinated peripheral nerves called Aδ fibers at about 6 to 30 m/s; this produces a pain response in approximately 0.1 second. Fast pain is usually described as sharp, pricking, or electrical.[14]

Slow pain impulses are carried from the periphery on smaller, unmyelinated fibers known as type C fibers. The speed of transmission ranges from 0.5 to 2 m/s. In these nerves, the pain response occurs in approximately 1 second or greater and can be more sustained. The clinical quality of this pain has often been referred to as burning, aching, throbbing, or nauseating.[14]

Excitation of nociceptors is produced by mechanical, thermal, and chemical stimulation. Chemical stimulation is related to substances such as bradykinin, histamine, serotonin (5-hydroxytryptamine; 5-HT), proteolytic enzymes, acids, potassium ions, and acetylcholine. In the periphery, other substances, namely substance P and prostaglandins, sensitize the receptors lowering the excitation threshold for stimulation by these chemicals.

Pain from ischemic tissues is caused by the release of chemical substances responsible for nociceptor excitation. An important clinical correlation is pain from muscle spasm. Pain is likely initiated by both mechanoreceptors at the site of spasm and chemical stimulation by the decreased blood flow caused by excessive muscular contraction.

From the periphery, neural stimulation is transmitted to the spinal cord and brain stem, then up through the brain stem to the thalamus, basal areas of the brain, and finally to the somatosensory cortex. Along these tracts, neural transmission is conveyed to various regions within the CNS where the nociceptive stimulation is processed and the beginning of the pain response begins. In addition, these pathways allow the neurotransmission received from the periphery to be regulated, modulated, or inhibited. It is at these levels that affective (emotional) and cognitive (thought) input is incorporated, helping to shape the pain response.

It is important to understand that nociception is not synonymous with pain. Nociceptors produce a signal, and the pain response requires that these neural signals be processed and receive important inputs from within multiple levels of the brain. This scenario is analogous to a power cord from an electrical outlet to a hand-held video game. The power cord delivers the electrical current but this current is processed by several components to create a display with lights and sound.

For patients, the clinical output after processing of nociceptive signals is the pain response. The pain response may be expressed in 2 ways: the external, objective expression of pain (pain behavior) and the subjective expression of pain (suffering).[15] Central to understanding the clinical implications of pain, especially chronic pain, is recognition of these variables in the pain response.

This classic pain model is useful in understanding acute pain and provides a platform for treatment strategies aimed at acute pain. However, this model does not explain all clinical pain responses, and the neurophysiology of chronic pain often has important clinical differences. In chronic pain conditions, changes within CNS pathways are at play. One example is central sensitization, which is an acquired condition within the CNS resulting from repetitive nociceptive stimulation from the periphery. Peripheral C fibers release glutamate in the spinal cord as their neurotransmitter. There are 3 subtypes of glutamate receptors in the spinal cord: kainate/AMPA (l-amino-3-hydroxy-5-methylsoxasole-propionic

acid,) NMDA (N-methyl-D-aspartic acid), and metabotropic subtypes. With persistent or large-scale activation of AMPA receptors, the NMDA receptor becomes activated and enhances all sensory inputs. In addition, NMDA receptor up-regulation induces apoptosis of neurons within the spinal cord with remodeling and formation of new connections. These new connections are devoid of μ-opiate receptors, making these nerves resistant to opiate/opioid treatment.[16,17]

Central sensitization is one example of neuroplasticity, which refers to changes that occur within the CNS in response to various stimuli or when somatosensory inputs have been altered. Such changes have also been shown to affect the trigeminal system.[18] Under these conditions, chronic pain may be a CNS response rather than a result of peripheral nociceptive signaling. As such, treatments that focus on peripheral conditions, as in the acute pain model, will be ineffective.

PAIN TERMS AND CLASSIFICATIONS

The International Association for the Study of Pain (IASP) defines pain as: "…an unpleasant sensory and emotional experience associated with actual or potential tissue damage or described in terms of such damage." As pointed out by Johnson in 1997, this definition considers the 3 important experiences that are associated with all forms pain: sensory disturbance, emotion (affective), and thoughts (cognitive). Additional characterizations of pain noted in the literature include transient pain, phasic pain, acute pain, and chronic pain.[19–21]

Transient pain is described as pain of brief duration and little consequence. Transient pain may be experienced after application of a noxious stimulus that produces minimal or no tissue damage. Examples cited are the discomfort experienced during venipuncture or when stubbing a toe. With minimal tissue damage, the pain sensation subsides quickly and there is rarely any need for medical attention. The function of the transient pain is thought to be injury prevention by activation of withdrawal and protective responses.

Phasic pain is of short duration and suggests that an injury has had an immediate impact. Phasic pain often involves reactions from the patient such as reflexive withdrawal from the stimulus, expressive behaviors that are recognizable as pain to an onlooker, nonverbal reactions, and protective movements.[22]

Acute pain can be defined as the experience caused by tissue damage, or impending tissue damage, and comprises a phasic state followed by a tonic state that will persist until healing takes place. As such, the pain will subside with resolution of the injury or condition that produces the pain. Acute pain is also often associated with a well-defined and clinically apparent cause, and is a protective reflex provoking withdrawal or escape from tissue stress and injury.[23] Acute pain can also aid the healing of injured tissue. By making that tissue sensitive to external stimuli, such as movement or touch, it will be protected and subject to fewer stresses. An example of this is the acutely sprained joint that responds poorly to movement and loading. Pain plays an important role, forcing decreased movement and loading on the joint and thus provides time for the healing process to proceed.[19]

For the oral and maxillofacial surgeon, the cause of acute pain is frequently evident. Surgical interventions are of primary importance in almost all of these situations including dental extraction, incision and drainage, curettage, reduction and fixation of fractures, and the administration of a local anesthetic injection. Within limits, the intensity and duration of the pain response in these daily clinical scenarios are predictable and, as such, are predictably managed. Treatments employed include procedural/surgical management of the noxious stimulus, the appropriate use of pharmaceuticals, and patient education and support, which will usually be very efficacious in managing the short-lived pain response.

What, then, is chronic pain? How does its management differ? Chronic pain has been defined in several ways usually with 2 constants: extended length of time and lack of ongoing tissue injury. One oft-quoted definition of chronic pain is "pain lasting for extended periods of time, lasting beyond the time needed for healing an injury. Frequently there may not be a clearly identifiable cause."[19] For the clinician who routinely manages acute pain, there may be an assumption that chronic pain is simply acute pain that is prolonged and not easily explained. However, along with its extended duration, chronic pain also is associated with an increasing likelihood of anxiety, depression, and social dysfunction as pain continues.[22,24]

Von Korff and Dunn[25] propose a prognostic approach to patients with prolonged pain. These investigators point out that "chronic" implies a state that is unlikely to change. Instead, chronic pain should be viewed as a condition that is fluid and has a great likelihood for change. When considering chronic pain in this light, treatment options exist and appropriate treatments will likely be efficacious. Von Korff and Dunn further write: "by shifting the focus from pain duration to prognosis... the assessment of chronic pain may be refocused from labeling patients... to focusing on steps that might be taken to reduce risks of an unfavorable outcome."

FROM THEORY TO PRACTICE

Clinicians are confronted with an array of terms and classification systems used to record and monitor their patients' pain experience. Within the oral and maxillofacial surgery literature, excellent reviews of facial pain classifications are presented.[1,7,8,26–28] An understanding of these terms and categorization systems of the pain experience are essential for proper diagnosis and management.

A useful method for documenting the patient's pain experience is the use of subjective descriptors elicited during history taking and responses seen with neurosensory testing during examination. Qualities such as sharp, dull, burning, throbbing, along with duration, onset, and relieving factors are well understood by doctor and patient.

Terms such as allodynia, anesthesia dolorosa, causalgia, dysesthesia, hyperalgesia, hyperesthesia, hyperpathia, neuropathic pain, and neurogenic pain are used to qualify pain and help develop a differential diagnosis. A thorough review of the definitions of these terms can be found in many sources, including the Web site for the IASP at www.iasp-pain.org.[29]

Okeson reviewed the classification of orofacial pain with respect to the type of tissue responsible for originating the nociceptive stimulation. He described somatic pain and neuropathic pain; the former arises from anatomic structures and tissues other than nerves whereas neuropathic pain arises from the neural structures themselves. Pain from somatic structures is further classified as superficial somatic pain, deep somatic pain, and visceral pain. The superficial somatic structures include cutaneous and mucogingival tissues. Deep somatic structures include musculoskeletal tissues, tissues of the temporomandibular joint, bone and periosteum, soft connective tissue, and the periodontium. Visceral structures include the dental pulp, vascular structures, visceral mucosal, glandular tissues, ocular tissues, and/or auricular tissues.[7]

In another article, Okeson[3] reviewed the concept of using a 2-axis system when evaluating patients experiencing pain. Axis I encompasses the physical factors at the proposed site(s) of pain and includes all of the classification systems described earlier. Axis II involves psychological factors. When evaluating any pain disorder both axes must be considered, as treatment addressing only one axis has a high likelihood for failure. Of course, patients with acute pain most often respond well with therapy directed at Axis I. In these instances, the pathology is causing an acute significant inflammatory response and treatment that will eliminate the pathology and reduce the inflammation (tooth extraction, pulpal extirpation, incision and drainage, fracture reduction, antibiotic administration, and so forth) should have a dramatic impact on reducing the patient's pain. However, as the pain experience becomes chronic, elevating the likelihood for concomitant anxiety, depression, and other psychological influences, Axis II factors must be addressed. For successful management of chronic pain, both axes require proper diagnosis and management.

Another important clinical distinction is whether chronic pain is associated with a malignancy. Chronic pain not associated with a malignancy is referred to as chronic noncancer pain (CNCP). Chronic pain secondary to malignancy is classified separately because cancer mechanisms causing pain are different from other chronic pain conditions. Although complex and variable, malignancies often produce ongoing destruction of tissue and thereby produce ongoing noxious stimulation. In CNCP, clinically apparent nociceptive stimulation or destruction of tissue may be absent. These 2 distinct categorizations of chronic pain are especially important in pharmaceutical management and are reviewed later in this article.

CAUSES OF CHRONIC PAIN CONDITIONS IN ORAL AND MAXILLOFACIAL SURGERY

Any injury that produces acute pain, whether surgical or traumatic, has the potential to evolve into a chronic pain condition. Fortunately, this is a rare occurrence in oral and maxillofacial surgery considering the number of procedures performed. In fact, when patients have pain that persists beyond the expected time interval for a particular procedure/condition, the search for a local pathologic cause takes precedent. For example, pain that persists in the mandibular third molar extraction socket that otherwise appears to be healing may be related to a bony sequestrum, an occult fracture, or the early stages of osteomyelitis. However, if symptoms continue after thorough serial evaluations and after exhausting all treatments for potential local pathology, a chronic pain condition must be considered.

Some of the more common conditions oral and maxillofacial surgeons encounter in patients who suffer from chronic pain conditions include pathology of the temporomandibular joint and temporomandibular disorders, head and neck malignancies, iatrogenic and traumatically induced nerve injuries, facial bone fractures, traumatic soft tissue injuries, burning mouth syndrome, trigeminal neuralgia, and other neuropathic conditions.

TREATMENT OF PATIENTS WITH CHRONIC PAIN

Before initiating treatment, a thorough history and physical examination is essential. Because chronic pain conditions are often not associated with clear-cut physical findings, the history takes on an even more critical role, and adequate time for this portion of the patient encounter must be provided. Allowing patients to describe their symptoms in their own words is important, and when needed, they can be helped with open-ended questions. In an effort to quantify patient symptoms, several scientifically validated pain questionnaires are available.

Even though chronic pain conditions often fail to manifest clear physical findings such as those seen in acute pain states, a thorough physical examination is essential. In fact, a skillful physical examination may uncover a pathologic condition that, when treated, might eliminate the patient's symptoms. Examples are a previously undiscovered carious lesion producing symptoms similar to atypical facial pain, or an undiagnosed nasopharyngeal or hypopharyngeal tumor causing unexplained otalgia or temporomandibular joint pain. The physical examination should also focus on changes that may be sequelae of the chronic pain condition. Examples are incisal/occlusal attrition and masseteric hypertrophy as a consequence of clenching and bruxism, mucosal trauma in an area of altered sensation following nerve injury with resultant neuropathic pain, and failed extensive dental treatment in a patient with symptoms of atypical facial pain.

Along with the physical examination are directed radiological and laboratory studies. Again, keeping in mind the need to rule out odontogenic sources of pain, a thorough radiographic survey of the teeth, periodontium, and maxillomandibular complex is warranted.

Even with ample data, an obvious diagnosis is often elusive in chronic pain conditions. Therefore, a carefully considered differential diagnosis should be developed. Along with Axis I maxillofacial diagnoses, potential Axis II diagnoses should be considered as well. These diagnoses will often be refined, or even changed, once the patient's response to treatments is assessed.

Finally, treatment may be prescribed based on the differential diagnoses. In the management of patients with chronic pain conditions, consideration should be given to each of the following elements: maxillofacial treatment, pharmaceutical administration, psychological intervention, and manipulative therapies. The order and weight of each element must be individualized for each patient. Also, just as vigilant monitoring of the patient's responses to treatment may refine or alter the diagnoses, treatment must also remain fluid. Strict treatment regimens that do not adjust to the needs of the patient are likely to be less efficacious.

MAXILLOFACIAL INTERVENTIONS

The oral and maxillofacial surgery literature is replete with medical and surgical strategies for the management of patients with chronic pain of the orofacial region. It is beyond the scope of this article to review specific surgical procedures. However, for all interventions, reasonable treatment goals should be developed. All prescribed treatment should attempt to achieve objectives in support of the goals. In patients with acute pain, this is usually clear: pathology is diagnosed, directed treatment is performed, followed by recovery and healing, then progress in a predictable fashion. With chronic pain conditions it may be challenging to align patient expectations with the likely outcomes of therapeutic interventions. Goals for treatment must be clearly defined and reviewed thoroughly with the patient. Given the prevalence of psychological issues in these patients, it is advisable to assess and perhaps address these before initiating surgical therapy.

PHARMACOLOGIC MODALITIES FOR CHRONIC PAIN MANAGEMENT

Pharmacologic management of pain continues to evolve as a consequence of the successes neuroscience has achieved in expanding our understanding of pain. As with other clinical conditions, pharmacotherapy attempts to target the suspected cause of each patient's pain experience. Contemporary pharmacologic paradigms take "aim" at various levels of the peripheral and central nervous systems and do so with a wide array of medications combined with various administration strategies—systemic, regional, local, and topical.[30–37] For chronic pain conditions, pharmacologic intervention is not limited to prescribing traditional analgesics based solely on an assessment the likely intensity of the patient's pain experience. Once again, the importance of multimodal treatment of patients experiencing pain cannot be overemphasized. The maximum

effectiveness of pharmacotherapy is dependent on its successful integration with other treatment modalities reviewed here.

The aim of this section is to review the pharmacologic management of chronic pain conditions. Chronic pain management is typically separated into 2 major categories, chronic noncancer related pain (CNCP) and chronic cancer pain. The management of chronic cancer pain is guided by the World Health Organization's (WHO) pain ladder.[30,31] Although this is a well-established tool, the management of chronic cancer pain is also influenced by individual patient needs and responses. The management of CNCP is not as structured. However, recent guidelines were published by the American Society of Interventional Pain Physicians and by the American Pain Society in collaboration with the American Academy of Pain Medicine to assist clinicians with the management of CNCP.[32,33] This review contains elements from these guidelines.

Nonopioid Analgesics

Acetaminophen inhibits prostaglandin synthesis centrally and therefore is not considered an anti-inflammatory agent. It is a relatively safe and effective analgesic for mild to moderate pain, both acute and chronic. Acetaminophen is considered the first-line therapy for symptomatic osteoarthritis, a noninflammatory arthritis.

Acetaminophen is commonly used in combination with opioids. Despite this, clinicians should not underestimate the analgesic efficacy of acetaminophen. Studies have shown little difference in pain control with acetaminophen alone verses a combination of acetaminophen with low-dose opioids, suggesting the majority of pain relief from the combination products is due to the acetaminophen component.[38]

Unfortunately, the risk of acetaminophen-related hepatotoxicity remains. Two areas of concern have recently been identified and reported by the Food and Drug Administration (FDA). The first concern is the excessive consumption of acetaminophen. In many cases, patients are unaware they are exceeding the recommended dose of acetaminophen. Patients should be educated about nonprescription products containing acetaminophen, warned of the danger of the self-administration of acetaminophen when taking opioid-acetaminophen combination analgesics, and advised not to exceed the prescribed dose of a combination product.[39–41] It is imperative that clinicians inquire about nonprescription medications and that they are aware of the doses of acetaminophen in the combination analgesics they prescribe. The second area of concern is the concomitant consumption of alcohol and acetaminophen, a combination that associated with an increased risk of hepatotoxicity.

These 2 issues led to the establishment in 2009 of an FDA advisory committee on acetaminophen.[39,40] This committee made several recommendations in an effort to reduce the incidence of acetaminophen-induced hepatotoxicity. First, the maximum daily dose of acetaminophen in a healthy adult has been reduced from 4 g to 3.2 g. Also, it is now recommended a single dose should exceed 650 mg. Another major recommendation was to require specific labeling of the packaging of acetaminophen-containing products in an attempt to increase public awareness of acetaminophen-induced hepatotoxicity. The FDA is also evaluating the following acetaminophen-related issues: considering removal of acetaminophen from certain combination products, determining a safe daily dose in chronic liver disease, and reestablishing appropriate pediatric dosing.

Aside from hepatotoxicity, the less common but clinically relevant adverse effects of acetaminophen usage include nephrotoxicity, dyspepsia, and rash. Overdose, both intentional and unintentional, are common and treatable with *N*-acetylcysteine if recognized early enough after ingestion.[39–51]

Nonsteroidal anti-inflammatory drugs (NSAIDs) and cyclooxygenase-2 (COX-2) selective inhibitors are used for a variety of mild to moderate chronic pain conditions including musculoskeletal pain, low back pain, osteoarthritis, ankylosing spondylitis, rheumatoid arthritis, dental pain, and chronic headaches. NSAIDs are considered to be more useful than acetaminophen for musculoskeletal pain, likely due the anti-inflammatory properties of the NSAIDs.[52–54]

NSAIDs' main mechanism of action is related to the inhibition on the synthesis of prostaglandins through blocking the enzyme cyclooxygenase (COX). The 2 isoforms of COX that are inhibited by NSAIDs are cyclooxygenase-1 (COX-1) and COX-2. Inhibition of COX-1 leads to the common side effects of NSAIDs by blocking the production of protective prostaglandins needed in the gut, vascular system, and by platelets. COX-2 inhibitors were developed to in an effort to selectively block inflammatory prostaglandins.[37,52–64]

NSAIDs have various adverse effects on the gastrointestinal (GI) system such as gastric irritation, dyspepsia, GI bleed and, to a lesser extent, Stevens-Johnson Syndrome (SJS) and toxic epidermal necrolysis (TENS).[37,52–60] The risk of GI events related to NSAIDs is based on the medication's relative COX-1 inhibition, dose and duration, as well as patient factors including a history of GI bleed, age over 60 years, use of other known GI irritant medications such as corticosteroids, history of *Helicobacter pylori*, history of dyspepsia, cigarette smoking, and alcohol use. Other common adverse effects of NSAIDs include sodium retention and hyponatremia, hypertension, renal failure, platelet inhibition leading to bleeding, hepatic dysfunction, and CNS effects including dizziness, sedation, and confusion.

As has been widely published, COX-2 selective inhibitors, and to a lesser extent the NSAIDs, have been associated with an increased cardiovascular risk.[61,62,64] This adverse effect is correlated with both classes of medication; however, the risk varies with the agent selected. Celecoxib is currently the only available COX-2 selective inhibitor on the market in the United States. The lowest possible dose should be used to minimize the risk of cardiovascular events.

Acetaminophen and the NSAIDs, including COX-2 inhibitors, all reach a dose at which analgesia is maximal and increasing the dose of medication will not enhance the analgesic effect.[30,37,54,55,64] Due to this ceiling effect, these medications are typically used for mild to moderate pain. In patients with moderate to severe pain they may be used, but most often in conjunction with additional medications such as opioids.

Opioid Analgesics

Opioids are effective for numerous types of moderate to severe pain including chronic cancer pain, acute postoperative pain, neuropathic pain and, to a lesser extent, CNCP. Opioids do not have a ceiling effect and therefore can be titrated up to the dose the patients need to treat their pain or until the adverse effects occur.[30–34,37,65–70]

Chronic opioids are the mainstay of treatment of cancer-related pain but their use for CNCP remains controversial.[30–33,37] A short course of opioids may be tried initially in such patients, but the decision to continue with long-term opioids for CNCP should be based on individual patient response to the initial trial.[32,33]

There are 3 major opioid receptor subtypes, mu, kappa and delta. The common mechanism of action all the opioids have is the central action on the mu opioid receptor in the CNS. However, therapeutic and adverse effects occur by activation of all 3 types of opioid receptors.[30–34,37,65–70]

There are several adverse effects commonly associated with opioids including nausea and vomiting, constipation, sedation, cognitive impairment, respiratory depression, hyperalgesia, and pruritus. These side effects should be anticipated and managed whenever possible with non-pharmacologic and, if indicated, pharmacologic modalities. Adverse effects of opioids may be particularly problematic in patients with chronic pain conditions for whom treatment periods may be significantly extended.[30–34,65–71]

Aside from their therapeutic and the unwarranted effects already noted, the chronic use of opioids is associated with 4 important conditions with which the prescribing doctor must be familiar: tolerance, addiction, psychological dependence, and physical dependence.

Psychological dependence and addiction are described in terms of the pattern of drug use characterized by craving for and compulsive use of opioids beyond their therapeutic effect. Every effort should be taken to avoid psychological dependence and addiction.[30–34,65–68,72–74] Tolerance and physical dependence, however, are expected physiologic consequences of chronic exposure to opioid therapy. Tolerance is a predictable increase in the dose required to produce the same therapeutic effect over time. Physical dependence is an adaptive physiologic state that leads to withdrawal symptoms with abrupt discontinuation of the medication. These consequences of therapy must be considered; however, opioids should not be avoided in patients for whom they are indicated. Special considerations should be taken for patients using chronic opioids, particularly in the perioperative setting.[16,30–34,65–68,73–77]

Clinically there are several avenues available to help the clinician determine if a patient is a candidate for opioid therapy. First, the Web site www.painedu.org is an excellent resource in providing tools and guidelines. In addition, psychologists play a major and unique role in assessing and managing patients in whom long-term opioid use is contemplated, accomplished through a process of evaluation and follow-up known as opioid medication monitoring. Psychologists document changes in a patient's daily function and chart them alongside changes in their medication; hence demonstrating if function increases or decreases as the level of medication changes. This information helps prescribers justify the appropriate long-term use of opioid medications or, conversely, defend the reduction/deletion of opioids from an individual's medication regimen.

Adjunctive/Alternative Analgesics

Anticonvulsants

Anticonvulsant mediations are commonly considered first-line therapy for neuropathic pain. These agents may also be useful in other pain states such as chronic migraine. Newer agents including pregabalin, gabapentin, lamotrigine, topiramate, zonisamide, and oxcarbazepine have become more popular than the older anticonvulsants, carbamazepine and valproic acid, because of their more favorable side effect profile. The principal adverse effect of the newer anticonvulsants is sedation; however, they are also associated with less common but serious side effects such SJS and TENS.[30,34,37,78–80]

Antidepressants

Antidepressants, specifically tricyclic antidepressants (TCA) and selective serotonin reuptake inhibitors (SSRI), have been used for chronic headache prevention, and neuropathic and musculoskeletal pain. SSRIs generally have fewer serious side effects; however, they are not as effective as the TCAs. Other antidepressants such as bupropion and venlafaxine have also been used for neuropathic pain and have fewer side effects than the TCAs.[30,34,37,80,81]

α2-AGONISTS

α2-Agonists (clonidine, dexmedetomidine, tiazantidine) act centrally by blunting the effects of norepinephrine in the CNS. These agents are used for lower back pain, neuropathic pain, fibromyalgia, and chronic myofascial pain. Side effects commonly associated with these agents are hypotension and bradycardia. Abrupt withdrawal of α2-agonists is commonly associated with rebound hypertension and tachycardia.[37,80,82–85]

NMDA receptor antagonists

NMDA receptor antagonists are often used in opioid-resistant chronic pain. Ketamine, dextromethorphan, amantadine, and methadone all have NMDA receptor antagonist effects. Methadone is an opioid with NMDA receptor antagonism, making it an attractive agent for the management of chronic pain, particularly when other more traditional therapies have failed to provide relief. Methadone should be used with care, as the opioid conversion is dependent on many factors. Methadone can increase the QTc interval, so caution should be used with high doses and when it is used in conjunction with other medication that can increase the QTc interval, as this may lead to torsades de pointes. The intravenous formulation of ketamine can be compounded into an oral solution for use in outpatient treatment of chronic pain, and is particularly useful for patients with hyperalgesia with opioids.[30,34,37,70,80,86–89]

NMDA receptor antagonists are notorious for producing vivid nightmares, but otherwise have favorable side effect profiles. Ketamine's effect on increasing blood pressure and respiratory rate has been clearly documented.[34,37,70,87,88]

Centrally acting muscle relaxants

Muscle relaxants include several classes of medications and may be used to help manage specific symptoms. The mechanism of action for most muscle relaxants is not known, with the exception of benzodiazepines, which work as γ-aminobutyric acid (GABA) receptor agonists. The major side effect of most of the muscle relaxants is sedation; they also have the ability to produce tolerance, physical dependence, and psychological dependence.[34,37,90] In addition, benzodiazepines have been linked to "downhill spiral." Downhill spiral refers to the loss of functional capacity and a corresponding increase in depressed mood. This functional and emotional decline has long been implicated as a consequence of long-term opioid use; however, this association has largely been anecdotal. While investigating the "pain-opioid downhill spiral," Ciccone and colleagues[91] discovered that benzodiazepines, not opioids, were statistically responsible for the downhill spiral.

Medical marijuana

Medical marijuana (cannabis) may be an effective adjunctive therapy in the management of chronic headache, musculoskeletal disorders, neuropathic pain, and cancer pain. Although the exact mechanism of action is not known, there seems to be an additive or even synergistic effect when it is used in combination with other pain medications, leading to a reduction in the dose requirement of the primary therapy. There are several routes of administration into the systemic blood flow including, inhaled, oral, and sublingual routes.[92-101]

As of the writing of this article, cannabis is listed as a Drug Enforcement Agency Class I medication, and as such cannot be prescribed by most practitioners. At present, several states in the United States have legalized medical marijuana use by patients who are authorized to do so by their physicians. Distribution is dictated by local legislation. The indications for its use are also strictly regulated in these states.

PSYCHOLOGICAL INTERVENTIONS

The interplay of psychology and chronic pain is complex. However, there are a few key concepts that should be understood by the oral and maxillofacial surgeon. First, the experience of pain is derived from sensory, cognitive, and affective inputs.[19,21,22] Second, chronic pain is associated with an increasing likelihood of anxiety, depression, and social dysfunction over time.[22,24] As such, the pain experience is often related to the severity of the emotional distress, and interventions are more likely to be beneficial if attention is paid to emotional processing of the pain experience.[23] Therefore, recognition of possible coexisting psychological manifestations of chronic pain and timely referral to a mental health specialist are important actions of the oral and maxillofacial surgeon. This section briefly reviews psychological constructs used in clinical practice.[8]

Anxiety and a sense of loss of control contribute to patients' suffering and have a negative impact on the pain experience. Techniques used to reduce anxiety and to allow patients to participate in their own care have had positive effects on the pain experience.[23,102]

The degree to which patients focus attention on their condition contributes to the pain experience—the more focused, the more distressing the pain. Shifting attention away from symptoms, as in the use of distraction techniques, decreases pain.[23]

There is a causal relationship between chronic pain and depression. Some investigators have reported nearly 100% prevalence of depression in patients with chronic pain conditions. Depression can increase automatic hyperactivity (muscle tension), increase sensitivity to acute pain stimuli, magnify medical symptoms, and is associated with impairment and loss of function.[103]

Other comorbidities closely linked with chronic pain states include mood disorders, sleep disturbances, opioid dependence, perception alteration, and behavioral changes.[102,103]

As pointed out by Carlson,[8] patients with chronic pain conditions must be viewed differently to most patients who present to the oral and maxillofacial surgeon's office. The symptoms and physical conditions experienced by these patients develop and evolve into a complex of physical, emotional, social, behavioral, and psychological factors that are often maladaptive and affect every aspect of life. Because of this, management strategies will often require biologic and behavioral modalities; in other words, biobehavioral treatment.

Alongside the biobehavioral treatment model, cognitive-behavioral therapy (CBT) is often employed in the multimodal management of chronic pain conditions. These therapies are based on the following principles. People are active processors of information and do not react passively to events or physical inputs. Thought, or cognition, can modulate physiologic and affective responses, both of which can impact on behavior. Conversely, affect, physiology, and behavior can influence one's thinking process. In addition, behavior is determined by the environment and the individual, and people create their own reality. Therefore, just as patients have developed and maintained maladaptive thoughts, feelings, and behaviors, they can also be engaged to change these maladaptive modes to more adaptive ones.[104] Of the 3 aspects of pain, namely sensory, cognitive, and affective, CBT is directed at the cognitive and affective components.

The scope of these therapies is extensive and includes education, behavioral skills training, cognitive skills training, relaxation training, and motivation enhancement training.[8,104]

It is also essential that the oral and maxillofacial surgeon understand the impact of underlying psychological conditions on clinical outcome. Studies have shown that preexisting psychological conditions are actually predictive of developing chronic pain conditions. Furthermore, in certain types of surgery, psychological factors more accurately predict outcome over pretreatment physical findings and degree of altered function.[105] Hence, pretreatment psychological screening (as discussed by Lyne and colleagues in other articles in this issue) is necessary for optimal surgical and nonsurgical treatment outcomes.

MANIPULATIVE THERAPIES

Manipulative therapies consist of nonsurgical procedures employed to help treat and rehabilitate patients suffering from pain and dysfunction. Typical physical therapies employed include electrophysical agents such as transcutaneous electrical nerve stimulation, joint mobilization and manipulation, soft tissue massage, and exercise.[22] These manipulations may be performed by the oral maxillofacial surgeon or by specialists including dental professionals skilled in managing chronic facial pain conditions, physical therapists, massage therapists, and chiropractors. Other physical manipulations include acupressure and acupuncture.

Along with these physical modalities, cognitive behavioral therapies such as relaxation and imagery techniques can also be performed.[22] These therapies may work best when under the guidance of a psychologist.

SUMMARY

Pain is a clinical response determined by sensory input, which is processed in the CNS using emotional and cognitive modulation. With acute pain, the source of sensory input is usually evident. Eliminating or reducing the pathology contributing to nociceptive signals is the primary tenet in management of acute pain conditions. Concurrent pharmacologic intervention helps to reduce symptoms, while time resolves symptoms. Chronic pain, however, is not simply prolonged acute pain. With chronic pain conditions, neuroanatomic changes within the CNS, along with greater emotional and cognitive influences, provide different challenges for the treating clinician. Acute pain treatment paradigms are not effective in managing patients with chronic pain conditions.

Management strategies begin with a thorough history and physical examination. Pain assessment should include quality and quantity of pain as well as its influence on quality of life and its emotional/psychological impact. Pharmacologic interventions include classes of medications beyond the traditional "pain" medications. Long-term use of medications, including opioids, may be required. Opioid management may be conducted safely in conjunction with a psychologist using opioid medication monitoring. Additional vital roles of the psychologist includes performance of pretreatment assessments, quantification and qualification of psychological diagnosis, monitoring for "downhill spiral" seen in some patients on long-term opioids and benzodiazepines, and instituting therapy for the cognitive and emotional aspects of pain.

Lastly, the impact of manipulative therapies should not be underestimated. Many of these treatment modalities have been reviewed in the literature. The search for patient-specific treatments should remain the primary goal of all practitioners involved with the management of patients with chronic pain conditions.

REFERENCES

1. Merrill RL. Neurophysiology of orofacial pain. Oral Maxillofac Surg Clin North Am 2000;12(2):165–79.
2. Bodner S. Psychologic aspects of chronic pain. Oral Maxillofac Surg Clin North Am 2000;12(2): 181–203.
3. Okeson JP. The differential diagnosis of orofacial pains. Oral Maxillofac Surg Clin North Am 2000; 12(2):205–16.
4. Dionne RA. Pharmacologic treatment of acute and chronic orofacial pain. Oral Maxillofac Surg Clin North Am 2000;12(2):309–20.
5. Halpern LR, Ogle OE. Alternative treatment modalities for orofacial pain. Oral Maxillofac Surg Clin North Am 2000;12(2):321–34.
6. Crane MA, Green PG, Gordon NC. Pharmacology of opioid and nonopioid analgesics. Oral Maxillofac Surg Clin North Am 2001;13(1):1–13.

7. Okeson JP. The classification of orofacial pains. Oral Maxillofac Surg Clin North Am 2008;20(2): 133–44, v.

8. Carlson CR. Psychological considerations for chronic orofacial pain. Oral Maxillofac Surg Clin North Am 2008;20(2):185–95, vi.

9. Hersh EV, Balasubramaniam R, Pinto A. Pharmacologic management of temporomandibular disorders. Oral Maxillofac Surg Clin North Am 2008;20(2):197–210, vi.

10. Benoliel R, Eliav E. Neuropathic orofacial pain. Oral Maxillofac Surg Clin North Am 2008;20(2):237–54, vii.

11. Fischer DJ, Klasser GD, Epstein JB. Cancer and orofacial pain. Oral Maxillofac Surg Clin North Am 2008;20(2):287–301, vii.

12. Klasser GD, Fischer DJ, Epstein JB. Burning mouth syndrome: recognition, understanding, and management. Oral Maxillofac Surg Clin North Am 2008;20(2):255–71, vii.

13. Melzack R, Wall PD. Pain mechanisms: a new theory. Science 1965;150(699):971–9.

14. Guyton AC, Hall JE. Textbook of medical physiology. 11th edition. Philadelphia: Elsevier Saunders; 2006.

15. Turk DC, Okifuji A. Assessment of patients' reporting of pain: an integrated perspective. Lancet 1999;353(9166):1784–8.

16. Hansen GR. Management of chronic pain in the acute care setting. Emerg Med Clin North Am 2005;23(2):307–38.

17. Bennett GJ. Update on the neurophysiology of pain transmission and modulation: focus on the NMDA-receptor. J Pain Symptom Manage 2000; 19(Suppl 1):S2–6.

18. Gobel S. An electron microscopic analysis of the trans-synaptic effects of peripheral nerve injury subsequent to tooth pulp extirpations on neurons in laminae I and II of the medullary dorsal horn. J Neurosci 1984;4(9):2281–90.

19. Johnson MI. The Physiology of the sensory dimensions of clinical pain. Physiotherapy 1997;83(10): 526–36.

20. Kolt GS, Andersen MB. Psychology in the physical and manual therapies. New York. Edinburgh (UK): Churchill Livingstone; 2004.

21. Fields H. Depression and pain a neurobiological model. Neuropsychiatry Neuropsychol Behav Neurol 1991;4(1):83–92.

22. Kolt GS. Pain and its management. New York. In: Kolt GS, Andersen MB, editors. Psychology in the physical and manual therapies. Edinburgh (UK): Churchill Livingstone; 2004. p. 141–61.

23. Korol CT, Craig KD. Pain perspectives of health psychology and culture. In: Kazarian SS, Evans DR, editors. Handbook of cultural health psychology. San Diego: Academic Press; 2001. p. 241–64.

24. Craig KD. Emotional aspects of pain. In: Wall PD, Melzack R, editors. Textbook of pain. 3rd edition. Edinburgh (UK): Churchill Livingstone; 1994. p. 261–74.

25. Von Korff M, Dunn KM. Chronic pain reconsidered. Pain 2008;138(2):267–76.

26. LaBanc JP. Classification of nerve injuries. Oral Maxillofac Surg Clin North Am 1992;4(2): 285–96.

27. Cooper BY, Sessle BJ. Anatomy, physiology, and pathophysiology of trigeminal system paresthesias and dysesthesias. Oral Maxillofac Surg Clin North Am 1992;4(2):297–322.

28. Zuniga JR. Normal response to nerve injury: histology and psychophysics of degeneration and regeneration. Oral Maxillofac Surg Clin North Am 1992;4(2):323–37.

29. Part III: pain terms, a current list with definitions and notes on usage. In: Merskey H, Bogduk N, editors. Classification of chronic pain. 2nd edition. Seattle (WA): IASP Press; 1994. p. 209–14.

30. Maiskowski C, Cleary J, Burney R, et al. Guideline for the management of cancer pain in adults and children. APS clinical practice guideline series, vol. 3. Glenview (IL): American Pain Society; 2005.

31. World Health Organization. Cancer pain relief. Albany (NY). Geneva (Switzerland): World Health Organization; WHO Publications Center USA distributor; 1986.

32. Chou R, Fanciullo GJ, Fine PG, et al. Clinical guidelines for the use of chronic opioid therapy in chronic noncancer pain. J Pain 2009;10(2): 113–30.

33. Trescot AM, Helm S, Hansen H, et al. Opioids in the management of chronic non-cancer pain: an update of American Society of the Interventional Pain Physicians' (ASIPP) Guidelines. Pain Physician 2008;11(Suppl 2):S5–62.

34. Argoff CE. A focused review on the use of botulinum toxins for neuropathic pain. Clin J Pain 2002;18(Suppl 6):S177–81.

35. Cohen SP, Dragovich A. Intrathecal analgesia. Anesthesiol Clin 2007;25(4):863–82, viii.

36. Ghafoor VL, Epshteyn M, Carlson GH, et al. Intrathecal drug therapy for long-term pain management. Am J Health Syst Pharm 2007;64(23): 2447–61.

37. Dworkin RH, Backonja M, Rowbotham MC, et al. Advances in neuropathic pain: diagnosis, mechanisms, and treatment recommendations. Arch Neurol 2003;60(11):1524–34.

38. Li Wan Po A, Zhang WY. Systematic overview of co-proxamol to assess analgesic effects of addition of dextropropoxyphene to paracetamol. BMJ 1997; 315(7122):1565–71.

39. Department of Health and Human Services; Food and Drug Administration. Organ-specific warnings;

internal analgesic, antipyretic, and antirheumatic drug products for over-the-counter human use; final monograph. Final rule. Fed Regist 2009;74 (81):19385–409.

40. US Food and Drug Administration. Public health problem of liver injury related to the use of acetaminophen in both over-the-counter (OTC) and prescription (RX) products. 2009. Available at: http://www.fda.gov/AdvisoryCommittees/Calendar/ucm143083.htm. Accessed August 5, 2009.

41. James LP, Capparelli EV, Simpson PM, et al. Acetaminophen-associated hepatic injury: evaluation of acetaminophen protein adducts in children and adolescents with acetaminophen overdose. Clin Pharmacol Ther 2008;84(6):684–90.

42. Schmidt LE, Dalhoff K. Serum phosphate is an early predictor of outcome in severe acetaminophen-induced hepatotoxicity. Hepatology 2002;36(3):659–65.

43. Crowell C, Lyew RV, Givens M, et al. Caring for the mother, concentrating on the fetus: intravenous N-acetylcysteine in pregnancy. Am J Emerg Med 2008;26(6):735.e1–2.

44. Wolf SJ, Heard K, Sloan EP, et al. Clinical policy: critical issues in the management of patients presenting to the emergency department with acetaminophen overdose. Ann Emerg Med 2007;50 (3):292–313.

45. Betten DP, Cantrell FL, Thomas SC, et al. A prospective evaluation of shortened course oral N-acetylcysteine for the treatment of acute acetaminophen poisoning. Ann Emerg Med 2007; 50(3):272–9.

46. Dart RC, Erdman AR, Olson KR, et al. Acetaminophen poisoning: an evidence-based consensus guideline for out-of-hospital management. Clin Toxicol (Phila) 2006;44(1):1–18.

47. Chamberlain JM, Gorman RL, Oderda GM, et al. Use of activated charcoal in a simulated poisoning with acetaminophen: a new loading dose for N-acetylcysteine? Ann Emerg Med 1993;22(9): 1398–402.

48. Gardner CR, Heck DE, Yang CS, et al. Role of nitric oxide in acetaminophen-induced hepatotoxicity in the rat. Hepatology 1998;27(3):748–54.

49. Larson AM. Acetaminophen hepatotoxicity. Clin Liver Dis 2007;11(3):525–48, vi.

50. Perry HE, Shannon MW. Acetaminophen. In: Haddad LM, Shannon MW, Winchester JF, et al, editors. Clinical management of poisoning and drug overdose. 3rd edition. Philadelphia (PA): WB Saunders; 1998. p. 664–74.

51. Whyte IM, Francis B, Dawson AH. Safety and efficacy of intravenous N-acetylcysteine for acetaminophen overdose: analysis of the Hunter Area Toxicology Service (HATS) database. Curr Med Res Opin 2007;23(10):2359–68.

52. Vane JR, Botting RM. Mechanism of action of aspirin-like drugs. Semin Arthritis Rheum 1997; 26(6 Suppl 1):2–10.

53. Kaufmann WE, Andreasson KI, Isakson PC, et al. Cyclooxygenases and the central nervous system. Prostaglandins 1997;54(3):601–24.

54. Ong CK, Lirk P, Tan CH, et al. An evidence-based update on nonsteroidal anti-inflammatory drugs. Clin Med Res 2007;5(1):19–34.

55. de Leeuw PW. Nonsteroidal anti-inflammatory drugs and hypertension. The risks in perspective. Drugs 1996;51(2):179–87.

56. Hirschowitz BI. Nonsteroidal antiinflammatory drugs and the gastrointestinal tract. Gastroenterologist 1994;2(3):207–23.

57. Ward KE, Archambault R, Mersfelder TL. Severe adverse skin reactions to nonsteroidal antiinflammatory drugs: a review of the literature. Am J Health Syst Pharm 2010;67(3):206–13.

58. Schafer AI. Effects of nonsteroidal antiinflammatory drugs on platelet function and systemic hemostasis. J Clin Pharmacol 1995;35(3):209–19.

59. Herndon CM, Hutchison RW, Berdine HJ, et al. Management of chronic nonmalignant pain with nonsteroidal antiinflammatory drugs. Joint opinion statement of the Ambulatory Care, Cardiology, and Pain and Palliative Care Practice and Research Networks of the American College of Clinical Pharmacy. Pharmacotherapy 2008;28(6):788–805.

60. Castellsague J, Holick CN, Hoffman CC, et al. Risk of upper gastrointestinal complications associated with cyclooxygenase-2 selective and nonselective nonsteroidal antiinflammatory drugs. Pharmacotherapy 2009;29(12):1397–407.

61. Vardeny O, Solomon SD. Cyclooxygenase-2 inhibitors, nonsteroidal anti-inflammatory drugs, and cardiovascular risk. Cardiol Clin 2008;26(4): 589–601.

62. Grosser T, Fries S, FitzGerald GA. Biological basis for the cardiovascular consequences of COX-2 inhibition: therapeutic challenges and opportunities. J Clin Invest 2006;116(1):4–15.

63. Grosser T. The pharmacology of selective inhibition of COX-2. Thromb Haemost 2006;96(4):393–400.

64. Antman EM, Bennett JS, Daugherty A, et al. Use of nonsteroidal antiinflammatory drugs: an update for clinicians: a scientific statement from the American Heart Association. Circulation 2007;115(12): 1634–42.

65. Kahan M, Srivastava A, Wilson L, et al. Opioids for managing chronic non-malignant pain: safe and effective prescribing. Can Fam Physician 2006;52 (9):1091–6.

66. Savage SR, Joranson DE, Covington EC, et al. Definitions related to the medical use of opioids: evolution towards universal agreement. J Pain Symptom Manage 2003;26(1):655–67.

67. Nicholson B. Responsible prescribing of opioids for the management of chronic pain. Drugs 2003; 63(1):17−32.

68. Pyati S, Gan TJ. Perioperative pain management. CNS Drugs 2007;21(3):185−211.

69. Furlan AD, Sandoval JA, Mailis-Gagnon A, et al. Opioids for chronic noncancer pain: a meta-analysis of effectiveness and side effects. CMAJ 2006;174(11):1589−94.

70. Sandoval JA, Furlan AD, Mailis-Gagnon A. Oral methadone for chronic noncancer pain: a systematic literature review of reasons for administration, prescription patterns, effectiveness, and side effects. Clin J Pain 2005;21(6):503−12.

71. Angst MS, Clark JD. Opioid-induced hyperalgesia: a qualitative systematic review. Anesthesiology 2006;104(3):570−87.

72. Smith HS, Kirsh KL, Passik SD. Chronic opioid therapy issues associated with opioid abuse potential. J Opioid Manag 2009;5(5):287−300.

73. Hariharan J, Lamb GC, Neuner JM. Long-term opioid contract use for chronic pain management in primary care practice. A five year experience. J Gen Intern Med 2007;22(4):485−90.

74. Inturrisi C, Hanks GWC. Chapter 4.2.3. New York. In: Doyle D, Hanks GWC, MacDonald N, editors. Oxford textbook of palliative medicine. Oxford: Oxford University Press; 1993. p. 845, xv.

75. Patanwala AE, Jarzyna DL, Miller MD, et al. Comparison of opioid requirements and analgesic response in opioid-tolerant versus opioid-naive patients after total knee arthroplasty. Pharmacotherapy 2008;28(12):1453−60.

76. Trescot AM, Glaser SE, Hansen H, et al. Effectiveness of opioids in the treatment of chronic non-cancer pain. Pain Physician 2008;11(Suppl 2):S181−200.

77. Smith HS. Variations in opioid responsiveness. Pain Physician 2008;11(2):237−48.

78. Blommel ML, Blommel AL. Pregabalin: an antiepileptic agent useful for neuropathic pain. Am J Health Syst Pharm 2007;64(14):1475−82.

79. Rzany B, Correia O, Kelly JP, et al. Risk of Stevens-Johnson syndrome and toxic epidermal necrolysis during first weeks of antiepileptic therapy: a case-control study. Study Group of the International Case Control Study on Severe Cutaneous Adverse Reactions. Lancet 1999;353(9171):2190−4.

80. Lipman AG. Analgesic drugs for neuropathic and sympathetically maintained pain. Clin Geriatr Med 1996;12(3):501−15.

81. Mattia C, Paoletti F, Coluzzi F, et al. New antidepressants in the treatment of neuropathic pain. A review. Minerva Anestesiol 2002;68(3):105−14.

82. Byas-Smith MG, Max MB, Muir J, et al. Transdermal clonidine compared to placebo in painful diabetic neuropathy using a two-stage 'enriched enrollment' design. Pain 1995;60(3):267−74.

83. Zeigler D, Lynch SA, Muir J, et al. Transdermal clonidine versus placebo in painful diabetic neuropathy. Pain 1992;48(3):403−8.

84. Max MB, Schafer SC, Culnane M, et al. Association of pain relief with drug side effects in postherpetic neuralgia: a single-dose study of clonidine, codeine, ibuprofen, and placebo. Clin Pharmacol Ther 1988;43(4):363−71.

85. Szumita PM, Baroletti SA, Anger KE, et al. Sedation and analgesia in the intensive care unit: evaluating the role of dexmedetomidine. Am J Health Syst Pharm 2007;64(1):37−44.

86. Nesher N, Ekstein MP, Paz Y, et al. Morphine with adjuvant ketamine vs higher dose of morphine alone for immediate postthoracotomy analgesia. Chest 2009;136(1):245−52.

87. Grant IS, Nimmo WS, Clements JA. Pharmacokinetics and analgesic effects of i.m. and oral ketamine. Br J Anaesth 1981;53(8):805−10.

88. Kannan TR, Saxena A, Bhatnagar S, et al. Oral ketamine as an adjuvant to oral morphine for neuropathic pain in cancer patients. J Pain Symptom Manage 2002;23(1):60−5.

89. Friedman R, Jallo J, Young WF. Oral ketamine for opioid-resistant acute pain. J Pain 2001;2(1):75−6.

90. Toth PP, Urtis J. Commonly used muscle relaxant therapies for acute low back pain: a review of carisoprodol, cyclobenzaprine hydrochloride, and metaxalone. Clin Ther 2004;26(9):1355−67.

91. Ciccone DS, Just N, Bandilla EB, et al. Psychological correlates of opioid use in patients with chronic nonmalignant pain: a preliminary test of the downhill spiral hypothesis. J Pain Symptom Manage 2000;20(3):180−92.

92. Abrams DI, Jay CA, Shade SB, et al. Cannabis in painful HIV-associated sensory neuropathy: a randomized placebo-controlled trial. Neurology 2007;68(7):515−21.

93. Abrams DI, Vizoso HP, Shade SB, et al. Vaporization as a smokeless cannabis delivery system: a pilot study. Clin Pharmacol Ther 2007;82(5):572−8.

94. Ellis RJ, Toperoff W, Vaida F, et al. Smoked medicinal cannabis for neuropathic pain in HIV: a randomized, crossover clinical trial. Neuropsychopharmacology 2009;34(3):672−80.

95. Giuffrida A, Leweke FM, Gerth CW, et al. Cerebrospinal anandamide levels are elevated in acute schizophrenia and are inversely correlated with psychotic symptoms. Neuropsychopharmacology 2004;29(11):2108−14.

96. Papanastassiou AM, Fields HL, Meng ID. Local application of the cannabinoid receptor agonist, WIN 55,212-2, to spinal trigeminal nucleus caudalis differentially affects nociceptive and non-nociceptive neurons. Pain 2004;107(3):267−75.

97. Wallace M, Schulteis G, Atkinson JH, et al. Dose-dependent effects of smoked cannabis on

capsaicin-induced pain and hyperalgesia in healthy volunteers. Anesthesiology 2007;107(5): 785–96.

98. Wilsey B, Marcotte T, Tsodikov A, et al. A randomized, placebo-controlled, crossover trial of cannabis cigarettes in neuropathic pain. J Pain 2008;9(6):506–21.

99. Noyes R Jr, Brunk SF, Baram DA, et al. Analgesic effect of delta-9-tetrahydrocannabinol. J Clin Pharmacol 1975;15(2–3):139–43.

100. Noyes R Jr, Brunk SF, Avery DA, et al. The analgesic properties of delta-9-tetrahydrocannabinol and codeine. Clin Pharmacol Ther 1975;18(1): 84–9.

101. Johnson JR, Burnell-Nugent M, Lossignol D, et al. Multicenter, double-blind, randomized, placebo-controlled, parallel-group study of the efficacy, safety, and tolerability of THC: CBD extract and THC extract in patients with intractable cancer-related pain. J Pain Symptom Manage 2010;39 (2):167–79.

102. Hansen GR, Streltzer J. The psychology of pain. Emerg Med Clin North Am 2005;23(2):339–48.

103. Fishbain DA. Approaches to treatment decisions for psychiatric comorbidity in the management of the chronic pain patient. Med Clin North Am 1999;83(3):737–60, vii.

104. Okifuji A, Ackerlind S. Behavioral approaches to pain management. In: Girard-Powell V, editor. Perioperative nursing clinics, vol. 4. Philadelphia (PA): Elsevier Inc; 2009. p. 317–26.

105. Celestin J, Edwards RR, Jamison RN. Pretreatment psychosocial variables as predictors of outcomes following lumbar surgery and spinal cord stimulation: a systematic review and literature synthesis. Pain Med 2009;10(4):639–53.

Occupational Stress in Oral and Maxillofacial Surgeons: Tendencies, Traits, and Triggers

Lauren D. LaPorta, MD[a,b,c,d,e,*]

KEYWORDS

• Stress • Burnout • Oral surgery • Dentistry

No aspect of life is more stressful and has more impact on overall health and well-being than occupational or job related stress.[1] This fact should not be surprising, considering the importance of work to human existence. Work provides a purpose and is closely associated with personal identity and one's role in society. It provides not only a means of financial support but also personal satisfaction. In the United States, the number of workers reporting that they were under high levels of stress more than doubled between 1985 and 1990.[2] The United Nations has called occupational stress "The 20th Century Disease" and the World Health Organization recognizes job-related stress as a worldwide epidemic.[3] The occupational characteristics most closely associated with the development of stress, burnout, and health-related difficulties are job demand, the degree of control in one's job, and social support at work.[4] Occupational stress is complex, involving more than one of these aspects working synergistically, such as time stress in combination with a perceived threat, high job demand, and low job control.[5,6] These situations predict a high incidence of physical and emotional illness, with the most hazardous combination being that of high job strain with low levels of social support.[6] It is this set of conditions that have been most highly associated with cardiovascular disease, musculoskeletal disorders, absenteeism, and poor quality of life.[4] There is also a high variability in individual responses to the same stressors and it has been theorized that individual characteristics such as coping style and personality traits have more effect than the nature of the job itself.[1,7] Although there are some stresses inherent to the nature of a given job, the effect varies depending on the individual performing the task. Thus, the stress experienced by a given individual in a situation is highly dependent on individual traits, tendencies, and triggers. The key to effective stress management lies in self-awareness and recognition of circumstances that lead to stress in the individual. Learning to identify sources of stress and become empowered to change or modify stressors is the most effective weapon in reducing and minimizing stress. Stress may be inevitable but it can be controlled.

Although stress is an issue for all workers, owing to factors inherent to care-giving work, it is more prevalent in the health professions. The dangers of stress to medical professionals have been a topic of discussion for more than 5 decades.[8] Dentistry has been further singled out as the health care field at even more risk for stress and related problems. Despite a vast body of literature, little progress has been made in identifying, treating, or preventing these disorders, and although oral and maxillofacial surgery (OMS) has been

[a] Department of Psychiatry, St Joseph's Healthcare System, 703 Main Street, Paterson, NJ 07503, USA
[b] Mt Sinai School of Medicine, 1 Gustave L. Levy Place, PO Box 1217, New York, NY 10029, USA
[c] Department of Medicine, Seton Hall University School of Health and Medical Sciences, 400 South Orange Avenue, South Orange, NJ 07079, USA
[d] Department of Psychiatry, University of Medicine and Dentistry of New Jersey-New Jersey Medical School, 185 South Orange Avenue, PO Box 1709, Newark, NJ 07101, USA
[e] Department of Psychiatry, St George's University, University Center, Grenada, West Indies
* Department of Psychiatry, St Joseph's Regional Medical Center, 703 Main Street, Paterson, NJ 07503.
E-mail address: laportal@sjhmc.org

Oral Maxillofacial Surg Clin N Am 22 (2010) 495–502
doi:10.1016/j.coms.2010.07.006
1042-3699/10/$ — see front matter © 2010 Elsevier Inc. All rights reserved.

identified as the most stressful and demanding of all dental subspecialties,[9] there is little literature that specifically explores these issues in OMS. One recent study found that nearly two-thirds of oral and maxillofacial surgeons worked in unsatisfactory conditions, predisposing them to high levels of stress and occupational dissatisfaction.[10,11] Areas of significant importance to dental specialists are management of professional and personal time and professional respect and standing.[12,13]

This article describes the basic concepts of occupational stress and burnout, discusses how dental professionals are affected, and considers how occupational stress and burnout may relate specifically to OMS. Finally, suggestions for identifying and managing stress are addressed.

STRESS AND BURNOUT: BASIC CONCEPTS

Stress, in the broadest sense, is a reaction to the demands being made on an individual. This definition does not automatically equate to a negative outcome. Indeed, some stress is positive and is necessary for survival as in the fight or flight response to a life-threatening event. When the demands of the situation exceed the individual's ability or capacity to handle them appropriately, the result is negative. Occupational stress is a complex condition and is described as the sum of the physical, mental, and psychological responses to work that are transformed into negative emotional reactions. Occupational stress may result in increased absences and decreases in productivity and service delivery.[10,11]

Occupational stress can be considered as the result of the interactions between individuals and their environment. How individuals perceive the demands of their jobs, the degree of control they exercise over the job, and the amount of support they receive from coworkers and supervisors determine how much stress they experience. Demand in this conceptualization, refers to workload and the amount of responsibility inherent to a task. The personal demands of an individual for perfectionism, success, and achievement are not considered but may be of particular relevance to the oral and maxillofacial surgeon.[14,15]

The amount of control and autonomy one has over the duties of a job and how the duties are performed to completion are also significant factors in the experience of occupational stress. The amount of control individuals have over their jobs is a function of their own needs for self-esteem and achievement. The ideal amount of control depends on the desires/needs of the individual and on personal career goals. Insufficient

control may lead to feeling undervalued and unappreciated; too much control, beyond which the individual feels comfortable, leads to feeling overloaded and overworked. When the control exceeds the individual's ability to cope, productivity decreases and stress increases. The final element, support, is inversely related to control: the more control one has, the less support that individual is likely to have in the workplace and the more they are looked to for providing support and leadership to other workers.[16]

The interactions of these 3 elements, namely, demand, control, and support, form the core of the demand-control model of stress (DCS). Jobs performed in conditions of low control and high psychological demand, predispose to adverse reactions and are harmful to health.[17] The risks for occupational stress are decreased when a balance is struck between the various dimensions of work and the needs of the individual. Individuals are in the best position to succeed when they have the optimal combination of what they need or expect from their work, what the work environment offers, and an effective interaction between the 2.[16]

A little stress may be healthy but constant overwhelming stress is not. Chronic stress metamorphoses into distress. The General Adaptation Syndrome model, proposed by Selye, describes 3 stages in the development of distress: alarm, resistance, and exhaustion. Initially, these responses are reactive and defensive. The individual recognizes that a stressful situation exists and begins to rally the appropriate defenses. If the stress continues unabated, the individual's defenses ultimately fail leading to a state akin to that of learned helplessness. Physical responses to stress that are, at first, beneficial to survival in the short term become pathologic and destructive if experienced chronically. The specifics and duration of this process in a given individual vary depending on the person's past experiences, inherent strengths, and vulnerabilities.[16] These individual variances are crucial to understanding how a person responds to a stressful situation. Psychological defense mechanisms, either gained from experience or taught, significantly affect an individual's physical response to stress.[18]

The experience of stress, then, is highly individualized. But the mind and body dyad does not exist in a vacuum. It rather shares a dynamic interaction with the environment. This interaction may best be described in terms of fit between the person and the environment. This model is based on several assumptions: people have the capacity for rational decision making, individuals and environments vary in reliable ways, and conditions that favor congruence between individuals and their environment favor vocational success.[16] It is important to remember that this is a dynamic rather than a static interaction. Thus, it is not a matter of simply trying to fit the person to the environment but to work toward finding the right environmental conditions for the individual. Environments may both promote or defend against stress. Some individuals may flourish in an environment of constant change and uncertainty, whereas others may prefer a more predictable work setting. Individuals may be able to effect sufficient controls over the environment to enhance fit. Conversely, they may possess enough insight into their own strengths and vulnerabilities to select environments that are more conducive to their comfort and productivity.

At its most extreme, occupational stress that is chronic or poorly managed can lead to a syndrome of burnout. Burnout can be considered an occupational hazard for those in health care and service related fields. The pressures, particularly emotional pressure, of having to respond to constant demands from patients in a caring and understanding way can take its toll.[19] This is characterized by physical and emotional exhaustion, depersonalization (distancing from others and/or negative attitudes toward patients), and lack of personal achievement or realization.[20,21] Job strain, high number of patients, problems related to care delivery, and a sense of lack of support and value to one's work predispose an individual to depression, both directly and through the development of burnout.[22,23] Burnout has been alternately described both as a process and as a condition. It is insidious, often developing as an adaptation to short-term stress, which becomes ineffective and harmful over the long-term. What may begin as protective emotional distancing may transform itself into emotional exhaustion and callousness. The result is the transformation of a previously committed professional to one who is disengaged from his or her work.[22]

Strategies to increase work engagement may be effective at preventing burnout. This changes the focus from preventing negative outcomes (burnout) to increasing overall well-being. Whereas burnout is considered to result from cynicism and exhaustion, engagement is from vigor, dedication, and absorption.[24] Career expectations factor highly in this formulation with higher rates of burnout and professional dissatisfaction present in those professionals who had unrealistic beliefs about what real-world practice would involve. Professional education may provide a solid academic foundation but may be less effective in preparing students for the day-to-day demands of the job.[25] In at least one study, the incongruence between expectations and career perspectives was found to be more predictive of the development of symptoms of burnout than actual working conditions.[26] It is significant that dentists, as a group, tended to score higher on measures of dedication and absorption than standard norms. The job resources most valued were immediate results and aesthetics. Idealism, pride, and the delivery of effective patient care were also predictors of high levels of professional engagement.[27] It is possible, then, to combat the negative aspects of stress, with increased attention to the things that really matter most to the dental professional. By finding ways to enhance the positive aspects of the job and to better prepare trainees for the demands of real-world practice, dental practitioners, including specialists, may be able to derive more satisfaction from their work and, ultimately, provide improved patient care.

STRESS AND THE ORAL AND MAXILLOFACIAL SURGEON: TENDENCIES

The specialty of OMS requires more training than any other dental specialty, averaging 12 to 15 years of higher education. After this rigorous training program, the practitioner works with patients who are under extreme physical and emotional distress from pain, traumatic injury, disfiguring tumors, and facial deformities (both functional and aesthetic). Further, these patients, in addition to being in pain, are often extremely fearful of the procedures to which they are subjected.

How does the DCS model relate to the practice of OMS? One study showed that 28% of oral and maxillofacial surgeons experienced high demands and low levels of control in their jobs. The demands can be quantitative (hours or pace of work) or qualitative (role conflict), whereas control refers to one's ability to use intellectual skills and to have the authority to make decisions about how to perform the work. Oral and maxillofacial surgeons who experienced high demands were more likely to be older than 40 years and to report symptoms of fatigue, anxiety, depression, and physical illness.[10,11] These findings should not be surprising because individuals who enter this field demand a high degree of perfection in themselves. By pursuing success in a demanding field that requires a high degree of control, they place themselves in a position of low support. In addition, they may work in conditions of relative isolation, having little contact with other professionals. This combination is a setup for burnout.

Burnout may be a problem for more than 10% of dental practitioners.[28] One of the major contributing factors to the burnout syndrome is the individual's perception of whether or not a situation may be controlled.[21] As stated, there is much that an individual practitioner should be able to control. An examination of professionals in 3 different subspecialties, namely, orthodontics, restorative dentistry, and OMS, demonstrated that, of the 3, orthodontists suffered least from symptoms of depersonalization. Oral and maxillofacial surgeons and restorative dentists, however, did not fare as well. The reason for this difference was thought to be the variable degree of control and flexibility that these specialists have over their clinic schedules. Orthodontists are able to interrupt their work for an emergency, if need be and there is far less urgency to their procedures. The surgical specialties, however, are far more demanding of the practitioners' time; that is, once started, a procedure cannot be interrupted or postponed, thus increasing time pressures.[9]

However, the high levels of stress indicate that many do not realize that they do indeed have a significant locus of control. One Canadian survey found that the more dental practitioners felt that situations were out of their control, the more exhausted they felt.[21] In a totally exhausted state, one is unable to objectively review the situation and pursue opportunities for change. Identification of those sources of stress that are internal, that is, derived from the intrinsic personality traits of dentists themselves, and those that are external (such as difficult patients, third party insurance claims) provides a template for effective management of a healthy practice.[29] One of the most common mistakes (and the greatest source of stress and frustration) is the tendency to make the individual fit the situation rather than the other way around.

The factors involved in the practice of OMS should be considered first. Although most of the literature specifically references dentists, oral and maxillofacial surgeons also work in similar circumstances and, therefore, the findings may be quite applicable and relevant. The typical dental office is plagued by time pressures, high caseloads, issues with staff, poor working conditions, defective materials or equipment breakdowns, and the routine boring nature of the job.[30] The dental suite is filled with noise from drills and other equipment and the dentist is exposed to known hazards.[31] Dentists and oral and maxillofacial surgeons work long hours, often in small cubicles in relative isolation. They require visual acuity, and their work involves repetitive movement, static positions, and exertion of force.[32] All of these factors are fraught with ergonomic issues: static positioning causes spinal misalignment and unnatural curvature of the upper back and neck[30,31] and small instruments are grasped and manipulated for prolonged periods and vibrating hand tools are used, leading to a host of work-related musculoskeletal disorders such as tendonitis, bursitis, and carpal tunnel syndrome.[32] Although all of these factors are recognized as creating a less than optimal work environment, the tendency in most cases is to make the individual fit with the work rather than to alter the conditions in which the work is performed. The focus is often on the adaptability of the person rather than on making interventions to adapt to the environment, emphasizing an external locus of control. In most cases, this is ineffective and only adds to the ongoing frustration inherent to the situation. This lack of attention to ergonomic design leads to chronic painful conditions that are responsible for the early retirement of many dental professionals.[30,33] Instead, if one focuses on potential interventions in redesign of a task, work environment, work schedule, and opportunities for career development, this empowerment will lead to a more positive attitude and increase the sense of personal achievement.[7] It has been recognized as such a significant risk to dentists and oral surgeons that the US Air Force commissioned a study of the ergonomics of dentistry. Their findings yielded many recommendations for improvement including lighter-weight handles for dental instruments, automatic handpieces that are more pliable and easier to activate, the use of better magnification and lighting to improve neck posture and minimize eye strain, and greater attention to the layout of the operatory to optimize accessibility of tools while seated.[34]

Perhaps the most difficult aspect of practice for oral and maxillofacial surgeons is dealing with patients who are fearful of procedures.[35] This aspect sets oral and maxillofacial surgeons and dentists up for a major role conflict that may contribute greatly to their stress. Specifically, dentists enter the profession from the desire to take on the role of a benevolent healer but are perceived instead by their patients as inflicting pain and inspiring anxiety and fear.[36,37] Dentists and oral and maxillofacial surgeons may then perceive that their profession is not respected and is viewed negatively by the general population. Although this belief is largely inaccurate, it may be a leading contributor to job dissatisfaction and occupational stress.[38] Although the public may not feel overwhelmingly negative toward the profession as a whole, it is clear that many people dread having dental procedures performed. Few look forward to going to the dentist, but most realize the importance of dentistry to overall health maintenance. OMS procedures are often handled on an emergent basis and may be initiated by significant trauma involving a life-threatening injury or major disfigurement. The oral and maxillofacial surgeon, then, more than any other specialist in the dental field, must be prepared to deal with severely distressed and anxious patients. Arguably, OMS practitioners require more interpersonal skills than their colleagues in orthodontics or restorative dentistry.

The acute distress of a patient, often seen on an emergency basis, presents oral and maxillofacial surgeons with unique challenges. The oral and maxillofacial surgeons must first overcome issues related to interruptions in their schedule and must work even more diligently to not exacerbate the patient's pain. Patient dissatisfaction ranks as the most stressful situation encountered by dental professionals,[39] followed by situations involving patients who are anxious or uncooperative, who experience significant pain, who move in the chair, or who grab the dentist's hand.[40] And it is these individuals on whom oral and maxillofacial surgeons and dentists rely for their livelihood and economic survival, further reinforcing a sense of role ambiguity.[28,41] Role conflict, role ambiguity, and a high degree of responsibility for others are the 3 major sources of stress for a dental practitioner and are significant predictors of hypertension.[7]

Oral and maxillofacial surgeons may experience significant role conflict within the medical profession. Their training is unique, often including completion of dental and medical school programs as well as residency. This is little understood by the general public, who may not realize or appreciate this additional level of training and expertise. Practice management issues also weigh heavily on the dental practitioner. Many feel unprepared for this task, having had little practical instruction in business and economics in dental school.[39] Time management issues have been identified as a persistent stressor for dental practitioners.[42] Although professionals may learn ways of handling many of the stressors of practice through experience, time management issues seem resistant to improvement over time and remain a source of frustration.[43]

The practice of OMS may indeed be inherently stressful, but awareness and recognition of early warning signs may help to mitigate the impact of stress on health and overall functioning. When the key factors of occupational stress, namely, job demand, control, and social support, are considered with regard to the practice of OMS, opportunities for change can be identified. The job itself is highly demanding, requiring delicate and precision work. Yet, given that most oral and maxillofacial surgeons are also running their own businesses, they should derive a high degree of control. This ability to control some of their stress, particularly as it relates to scheduling, office setup and equipment, and management of support staff, should theoretically position the oral and maxillofacial surgeons to have a relatively low degree of stress. Overwhelmingly, the evidence shows just the opposite: dental professionals experiencing high levels of stress within their working lives are subject to feelings of low self-esteem, depression, and anxiety and have a higher rate of suicide than the general population.[38]

Stress is so pervasive in OMS and dentistry that it is not a matter of if these professionals experience serious stress but a matter of when and how.[44] And, in turn, it may be less a matter of how than who; that is, individual differences in coping and personality style may be even more important. These differences are apparent in trainees and early career dentists and contribute strongly to the degree of distress experienced by individuals. Dentists are 3 times more likely to report anxiety than other professionals and have a disproportionate rate of alcoholism, drug abuse, and divorce.[39] In one large study of 3500 dentists, 38% reported always or frequently feeling anxious. Another third of respondents reported exhaustion, and one-quarter complained of headaches and backaches, symptoms frequently associated with stress in the general population.[40]

In addition to emotional stress, dentists and oral and maxillofacial surgeons are not only subject to all of the health consequences of stress shared by the general population, including cardiovascular disease, but also suffer physical stresses from practicing their profession. In addition to the musculoskeletal disorders already mentioned, these health consequences include dermatitis[30,45] and visual problems.[35]

The consequences of stress are far-reaching. Stressed dental professionals are less effective in providing care to patients, experience higher rates of staff turnover, and are more prone to accidents. Dissatisfaction with one's job life spills over into one's home life, leading to family problems, divorce, and even more isolation. Stress affects not only the dentist but also the dentist's staff, patients, and family.[44] Chronic stress is associated with the development of major depressive disorder and dysthymia, a chronic mood state characterized by depression and poor functioning, feelings of inadequacy, and erosion of professional relationships. The resultant loss of colleagues, staff, and patients may drive the oral and maxillofacial surgeon further into a downward spiral.[46] Such professionals no longer derive satisfaction from their work and this dissatisfaction has been identified as a major cause of early retirement.[42] Health is affected, with dental practitioners having an incidence of high blood pressure that is 25% higher than in the general population, putting them at risk for cardiovascular disease and stroke.[28,38]

High levels of stress are associated with increased anxiety and depression. Dentists have been considered at higher risk for suicide than the general population. It has been argued that the connection is spurious, but studies that control for confounding variables continue to demonstrate a higher-than-average risk.[39,40,47]

ORAL AND MAXILLOFACIAL SURGEONS: TRAITS

Like all highly driven professionals, dentists have a set of traits that may make them more vulnerable to stress and, ultimately, to the burnout syndrome. It has even been theorized that dentists, as a group, may be more emotionally vulnerable than their peers in other health care fields.[38] Before they even enter into practice, they exhibit personality traits and individual tendencies that provide a perfect backdrop for severe stress. Dental professions may attract individuals who are highly compulsive, who have unrealistic expectations and extremely high standards of performance, often to an unnecessary degree, and who seek social approval and status.[43] Common terms used to describe dentists are authoritarian, conservative, inflexible, controlling, and perfectionist; all traits are commonly considered part of a type A personality.[48] This personality type is common in those who are highly driven, ambitious, and high achieving. These individuals are impatient and aggressive, and the more of these traits they display, the less they are able to cope with occupational stress.[27] Traits such as compassion and dedication, often thought to be highly desirable, tend to increase susceptibility.[49] A significant number of dental professionals from all specialties, including orthodontics and OMS, demonstrate traits of narcissism; borderline and obsessive compulsive personality disorders,[17] all associated with poor coping skills; and vulnerability to the effects of acute and chronic stress.

STRESS MANAGEMENT: KNOWING THE TRIGGERS

Professional practice leads to stress no matter how much one tries to prevent it. Proactive management of stress is a key to preventing the long-term ill effects of stress on health and well-being. Oral and maxillofacial surgeons can take simple steps to decrease their stress levels and increase their sense of control, peace, and well-being. Recognizing the symptoms and admitting there is a problem is a good first step. The earlier one comes to terms with stress, the less the damage, both psychologically and physically. Not all stress is necessarily bad. If stress in a situation is viewed as a measure of the challenges inherent to the task, then moderate amounts of stress arising from challenging demands may lead to creativity, satisfaction, feelings of achievement, and increased self-esteem. Early warning signs of inadequate levels of stress may be boredom or restlessness. If the situation persists, loss of direction and hopelessness may occur, giving way to depression and alienation over the long term. Excessive demands, beyond which the individual feels comfortable handling, lead to high arousal and tension. If unabated, anger and worry ensue, ultimately giving way to anxiety, depression, and exhaustion.[43] Recognition of the earliest signs of trouble and implementing prompt interventions can reverse a negative situation into a positive one. The first consideration may be to examine the fit between the individual and the situation. Many tend to force a fit rather than to explore opportunities for change. Nevertheless, this may be a successful strategy for those who are able to find ways of changing some aspects of a job. Some situations may not easily yield to change and individuals may have to be prepared to seek out a new practice opportunity. Although this is an extreme solution, it may be the most appropriate over the long term.

Effective time management is another important step. Oral and maxillofacial surgeons must take control of their time. Time management, both professional and personal, is highly associated with occupational stress and overall job satisfaction.[11,14] Therefore, taking charge of these issues and learning to handle them more effectively has a significant effect on overall well-being. Learning to delegate tasks, although difficult for highly compulsive individuals, is a necessary skill to master. One simply cannot and, furthermore, should not, do everything alone. The oral and maxillofacial surgeon can delegate some tasks, particularly those that are unfulfilling and uninteresting, to other staff, thereby eliminating a significant source of professional stress.[50] Another effective strategy is simply building emergency time into the daily schedule. This strategy serves to decrease or prevent the oral and maxillofacial surgeon from becoming overwhelmed.

Improvements to the environment also help to manage stress. Soothing colors for the office suite not only positively affect the attitude of the oral and maxillofacial surgeon but also help to put patients at ease. Attention should be given to the setup of office equipment to provide an optimal ergonomic fit to the oral and maxillofacial surgeon to increase both comfort and efficiency.[51,52]

Recognizing those areas that are within the individual control of the oral and maxillofacial surgeon is vital to stress management. Many professionals skip lunch, work through their lunch breaks, and fail to make time for vacations and continuing education. These strategies, rather than making for a more efficient and productive oral and maxillofacial surgeon, pave the way to burnout. Taking time to eat a meal without checking e-mail, returning calls, or doing paperwork is not wasted time but time well spent.[53] Relaxation techniques, both inside and outside the office, may make a world of difference to the day of a busy professional. Just a few minutes of quiet time, deep breathing, brief meditation, or even catnaps can significantly improve overall functioning, allowing the oral and maxillofacial surgeon to return to the job feeling revitalized and refreshed. Trudging through fatigue only exacerbates feelings of frustration and discontent.

It is also important to develop outside interests. Everyone needs a hobby, and the pleasure derived from partaking in such activities helps to improve general well-being and overall outlook on life. All work and no play may not necessarily make for a dull oral and maxillofacial surgeon but does make for an unhappy bored one.

SUMMARY

Occupational stress is common in health care professionals. Oral and maxillofacial surgeons are subject to stresses owing to the nature of their work and from predisposing characteristics that may have led them to choose their career. By recognizing the early warning signs of stress and taking control of modifiable sources of stress, both internal (individual responses to stress such as irritability, anxiety, and autonomic responses) and external (ergonomics and time management), oral and maxillofacial surgeons may be able to effectively manage or reduce their stress and prevent the long-term effects and the potentially career-ending consequences of unmitigated stress. Practical strategies include relaxation, career enrichment, and the pursuit of fulfilling nonwork-related activities.

REFERENCES

1. Atkinson W. Strategies for workplace stress. Risk and insurance. 2000. Available at: www.findarticles. com/p/aritcles/mi_.m0BJK/is_13_11/ai_66930268/. Accessed November 27, 2009.
2. Northwestern National Life Insurance Company. Employee burnout: America's newest epidemic. Minneapolis (MN): Northwestern National Life Insurance Company; 1991.
3. Job stress. Available at: http://www.stress.org/job. htm. Accessed November 12, 2009.
4. Rusli BN, Edimansyah BA, Naing L. Working conditions, self-perceived stress, anxiety, depression and quality of life: a structural equation modeling approach. BMC Public Health 2008. Available at: http://www.biomedcentral.com/1471-2458/8/48. Accessed November 27, 2009.
5. Stanton JM, Balzer WK, Smith PC, et al. A general measure of work stress: the stress in general scale. Educ Psychol Meas 2001;61:866–88.
6. Dollard MF, Winefield HR. A test of the demand-control/support model of work stress in correctional officers. J Occup Health Psychol 1998;3(3):243–64.
7. Schneiderman N, Ironson G, Siegel SD. Stress and health: psychological, behavioral, and biological determinants. Annu Rev Clin Psychol 2005;1:607–28.
8. Russek HI. Emotional stress and coronary heart disease in american physicians, dentists and lawyers. Am J Med Sci 1962;243(6):716–26.
9. Humphris GM, Lilley J, Branfield D, et al. Burnout and stress-related factors among junior staff of three dental hospital specialties. Br Dent J 1997;183:15–21.
10. Carneiro SCA, Vasconcelos BC, Nascimiento MMM, et al. Occupational stress among Brazilian oral-maxillofacial surgeons. Med Oral Patol Oral Cir Bucal 2009;14(12):e646–9.
11. Roth SF, Heo G, Varnhagen C, et al. The relationship between occupational stress and job satisfaction in orthodontics. Am J Orthod Dentofacial Orthop 2004;126:106–9.
12. Karasek RA, Theorell T. Healthy work: stress, productivity, and the reconstruction of working life. New York: Basic Books, Inc; 1990.
13. Tansey TN, Mizelle N, Ferrin JM, et al. Work-related stress and the Demand-Control-Support framework: implications for the P x E fit model. J Rehabil 2009. FindArticles.com. Available at: http://findarticles. com/p/articles/mi_m0825/is_3_70/ai_n6237490/. Accessed December 11, 2009.
14. Turner JA, Karosh RA Jr. Software ergonomics: effects of computer application design parameters on operator task performance and health. Ergonomics 1984;27:663–90.
15. Williams LJ, Anderson SE. Job satisfaction and organization commitment as predictors of

organizational citizenship and in-role behaviors. J Manag 1991;17:601–17.

16. Alaujan AH, Alzahem AM. Stress among dentists. Gen Dent 2004;52:428–32.

17. Martinez AA, Aytes LB, Escoda CG. The burnout syndrome and associated personality disturbances. The study in three graduate programs in dentistry at the University of Barcelona. Med Oral Patol Oral Cir Bucal 2008;13(7):E444–50.

18. Humphris G. A review of burnout in dentists. Dent Update 1998;11:392–6.

19. Cherniss C. Staff burnout: job stress in the human services. Beverly Hills (CA): Sage; 1980.

20. Ahola K, Hakanen J. Job strain, burnout, and depressive symptoms: a prospective study among dentists. J Affect Disord 2007;104(1–3):103–10.

21. Hakanen J. Job engagement and burnout. Psykologia 2002;37:291–301.

22. Gorter RC, Eijkman MA. [Career expectations and the type of dentists in the light of burnout]. Ned Tijdschr Tandheelkd 2002;109(6):212–6 [in Dutch].

23. Gorter RC, Albrecht G, Hoogstraten J, et al. Work place characteristics, work stress and burnout among Dutch dentists. Eur J Oral Sci 1998;106(6):999–1005.

24. Gorter RC, Te Brake HJ, Hoogstraten J, et al. Positive engagement and job resources in dental practice. Community Dent Oral Epidemiol 2008;36(1):47–54.

25. Osborne D, Croucher R. Levels of burnout in general dental practitioners in southeast England. Br Dent J 1994;177:372–7.

26. Wycoff SJ. An examination of what dentists already know about stress and burnout within dentistry. CDA J 1984;12:114–7.

27. Freeman R, Main JRR, Burke EJT. Occupational stress and dentistry: theory and practice part II assessment and control. Br Dent J 1995;178:218–22.

28. Litchfield NB. Stress-related problems of dentists. Int J Psycosom 1989;36(1–4):41–4.

29. Thornton LJ, Stuart-Buttle C, Wyszynski TC, et al. Physical and psychosocial stress exposures in US dental schools: the need for expanded ergonomic training. Appl Ergon 2004;35:153–7.

30. Valachi B, Valachi K. Preventing musculoskeletal disorders in clinical dentistry. J Am Dent Assoc 2003;134(12):1604–12.

31. Murtomaa H. Work-related complaints of dentists and dental assistants. Int Arch Occup Environ Health 1982;50:231–6.

32. Finsen L, Christian H, Bakke M. Musculoskeletal disorders among dentists and variety in dental work. Appl Ergon 1998;29:119–25.

33. Burke FJ, Main JR, Freeman R. The practice of dentistry: an assessment of reasons for premature retirement. Br Dent J 1997;182(7):250–7.

34. USAF Dental Investigative Services. Available at: http://www.brooks.af.mil/AL/AO/AOC/AOCD/dis-home.htm. Accessed December 14, 2009.

35. Freeman R, Main JRR, Burke FJT. Occupational stress and dentistry: theory and practice Part I recognition. Br Dent J 1995;178:214–7.

36. Cooper CL, Cartwright S. Healthy mind; healthy organization—a proactive approach to occupational stress. Hum Relat 1994;47(4):455–70.

37. Cooper CL, Mallinger M, Kahn R. Identifying sources of occupational stress amongst dentists. J Occup Psychol 1978;51:227–34.

38. DeMatteo MR, Shugars DA, Hays RD. Occupational stress, life stress and mental health among dentists. J Occup Organ Psychol 1993;66:153–62.

39. Bourassa M, Baylard JF. Stress situations in dental practice. J Can Dent Assoc 1994;60(1):65–7, 70–1.

40. Gale EN. Stress in dentistry. N Y State Dent J 1998;8: 30–4.

41. Walker JI. Stress of practice: it can be reduced. Dent Econ 1981;6:51–5.

42. Newton JT, Allen CD, Coates J, et al. How to reduce the stress of general dental practice: the need for research into the effectiveness of multifaceted interventions. Br Dent J 2006;200:437–40.

43. Rada RE, Johnson-Leong C. Stress, burnout, anxiety and depression among dentists. J Am Dent Assoc 2004;135:788–94.

44. Myers HL, Myers LB. "It's difficult being a dentist": stress and health in the general dental practitioner. Br Dent J 2004;197(2):89–93.

45. Ayers KMS, Thomson WM, Newton JT, et al. Self-reported occupational health of general dental practitioners. Occup Med (Lond) 2009;59:142–8.

46. Frey R. When professional burnout syndrome leads to dysthymia. J Can Dent Assoc 2000;66:33–4.

47. Stack S. Suicide risk among dentists: a multivariate analysis. Deviant Behav 1986;17:107–17.

48. Katz CA. Stress factors operating in the dental office work environment. Dent Clin North Am 1986;30 (Suppl 4):S29–37.

49. Pride J. Why some dentists burn out. J Am Dent Assoc 1991;122(6):73–4.

50. Cooper CL, Watts J, Kelly M. Job satisfaction, mental health and job stressors among general dental practitioners in the UK. Br Dent J 1987;162: 77–81.

51. Kroeger RF, Stevens DE, Vamosi SJ, et al. Designing the dental office for relaxation. Quintessence Int 1986;17(11):755–60.

52. Cutler M, Cutler J. Ergonomics for treatment room planning. Dentalpractice 1981;2(2):45–8.

53. Byers MM. Seven ways to prevent burnout. J Mich Dent Assoc 2008;90:28.

Psychological Issues in Sleep Apnea

Mansoor Madani, DMD, MD[a,b,c,*],
Farideh M. Madani, DMD[d],
Marcella Frank, DO, FCCP, DABSM[e]

KEYWORDS

- Sleep apnea • Sleep-disordered breathing • Depression
- Mood • Affective disorders

Approximately 1 in 5 people who suffer from depression also suffer from sleep apnea, and individuals with sleep apnea are 5 times more likely to become depressed. Patients suffering from obstructive sleep apnea (OSA) often present with a variety of symptoms including fatigue, sleepiness, depression, and insomnia. Some patients are easily agitated at work, and others cannot concentrate and perform at work or home. These symptoms can also undermine the individuals' relationships with their families and may ultimately limit the ability to enjoy life.

This article relates to the clinical practice of both sleep medicine and behavioral medicine. Many of the symptoms present in OSA are common with the findings of depression and other mood disorders. It is crucial to assess sleep disorders in patients diagnosed with depression. OSA might not only be associated with a depressive syndrome, but its presence may also be responsible for a patient's failure to respond to appropriate pharmacologic treatment. Furthermore, undiagnosed OSA might be exacerbated by adjunct medical treatments to antidepressant medications.

Increased awareness of the relationship between depression and OSA might significantly improve diagnostic accuracy and treatment outcomes for both disorders. In this review, important findings on OSA are summarized, common symptoms related to the association between depression and OSA are described, and the possible mechanisms by which these disorders interact are explored. Implications for clinical practice are discussed.

DEFINITION AND PREVALENCE OF OSA

OSA is by far the most common form of sleep-disordered breathing and is defined by frequent episodes of obstructed breathing during sleep. Specifically, OSA is characterized by sleep-related decreases, shallow breathing and hypopneas, or cessation of breathing (apneas). An obstructive apnea is defined as at least 10 seconds' interruption of oronasal airflow, corresponding to a complete obstruction of the upper airways despite continuous chest and abdominal movements, and associated with a decrease in oxygen saturation and/or arousals from sleep. An obstructive hypopnea is defined as at least 10 seconds of partial obstruction of the upper airways, resulting in an at least 50% decrease in oronasal airflow.[1–4]

[a] Department of Oral and Maxillofacial Surgery, Capital Health Regional Medical Center, 750 Brunswick Avenue, Trenton, NJ 08638, USA
[b] Oral and Maxillofacial Surgery, Temple University, 3401 North Broad Street, Philadelphia, PA 19140, USA
[c] Bala Institute of Oral and Facial Surgery, 15 North Presidential Boulevard, Suite 301, Bala Cynwyd, PA 19004, USA
[d] Department of Oral Medicine, Robert Schattner Center, University of Pennsylvania, School of Dental Medicine, 240 South 40th Street, Philadelphia, PA 19104, USA
[e] The Center for Sleep Medicine, Capital Health's Center for Sleep Medicine, 750 Brunswick Avenue, Trenton, NJ 08638, USA
* Corresponding author. Bala Institute of Oral and Facial Surgery, 15 North Presidential Boulevard, Suite 301, Bala Cynwyd, PA 19004.
E-mail address: drmmadani@gmail.com

Oral Maxillofacial Surg Clin N Am 22 (2010) 503–509
doi:10.1016/j.coms.2010.07.007

About 2% of women and 4% of men older than 50 years have symptomatic OSA. The most common complaints are loud snoring, disrupted sleep, and excessive daytime sleepiness (EDS). Patients with apnea suffer from fragmented sleep and may develop cardiovascular abnormalities because of the repetitive cycles of snoring, airway collapse, and arousal. Although most patients are overweight and have a short thick neck, some are of normal weight but have a small receding jaw.

Patients with OSA may have difficulty concentrating, difficulty in remembering factual data, become irritable or withdrawn, and find themselves losing interest in or deriving little pleasure from activities that were an integral part of their lives. These symptoms bear a striking similarity to some of those ascribed to depression and may potentially fulfill the criteria for a major depressive episode. Therefore, the potential certainly exists for misdiagnosis of OSA or depression. The other question is whether the presence of one of these conditions increases the likelihood of the other. Previous studies have identified an increased incidence of the symptoms of depression in patients with OSA and an increased incidence of the symptoms of OSA in patients with depression.[5–8]

However, other reports on the effectiveness of various measures to treat OSA and having positive results in alleviating symptoms of depression have provided mixed results.[9–15] Chronic sleep problems affect 50% to 80% of patients in a typical psychiatric practice, compared with 10% to 18% of adults in the general United States population. Sleep problems are particularly prevalent in patients with anxiety, depression, bipolar disorder, and attention-deficit/hyperactivity disorder.[16]

SHARED SYMPTOMS OF DEPRESSION AND OSA

Symptoms of both depression and sleep apnea vary from person to person; however, there are many symptoms shared by both. The following is a list of the most common symptoms. It should be noted that these symptoms may not be present in all patients:

- Daytime sleepiness
- Loss of energy
- Headaches
- Concentration impairment
- Forgetfulness and memory loss or lapses
- Impaired judgment
- Anxiety
- Irritability
- Loss of libido

- Changes in weight and appetite
- Insomnia
- Loss of interest in things that were once pleasurable
- Feelings of hopelessness, helplessness, and sadness.

The extent to which daytime functioning is affected generally depends on the severity of OSA. Symptoms other than EDS that greatly affect daytime functioning are neuropsychological symptoms such as irritability, difficulty concentrating, cognitive impairment, depressive symptoms, and other psychological disturbances. Thus, OSA can easily mimic symptoms of a major depressive episode.

Correlation Between OSA and Depression: Shared Risk Factors

Sleep disorders and insomnia traditionally have been recognized as symptoms of many psychiatric disorders. However, current studies in both adults and children suggest that sleep disorders may in fact be the cause or a major contributing factor for the development of some psychiatric disorders. The significance of this new understanding lies in the potential for successful treatment of OSA to alleviate symptoms of a comorbid mental health problem in some cases. A good night's sleep helps foster both mental and emotional resilience, whereas chronic sleep disruptions set the stage for negative thinking and emotional vulnerability.[17,18]

With all the common factors shared by depression and OSA in mind, several important assumptions can be developed. First, consider the cohort of patients with a definitive diagnosis of OSA, which is confirmed by clinical findings and various methods of polysomnography but misdiagnosed as having psychological issues. In these cases, the symptoms of depression should subside or be completely eliminated by using multiapproach techniques including nonsurgical treatments with continuous positive airway pressure (CPAP), bilevel positive airway pressure, demand positive airway pressure, or oral appliances and surgical treatments if indicated. Resolution of OSA in these patients may be brought about by eliminating upper airway obstructions, normalizing oxygen delivery to the patient, and eliminating sleep fragmentations.[19]

In a second group of patients, the obstructive respiratory events and the subsequent sleep fragmentation might have caused neurochemical alterations in the brain that result in depression. In these cases, the diagnosis of depression is assumed to be correct, but the underlying cause is attributed to OSA. It can then be assumed that treatment of the underlying cause of apnea might result in an improvement of the secondary syndrome of depression.[20–22]

A third group of patients suffers from 2 separate disorders but with similar underlying mechanisms. It is possible that the neurochemical aberration in the brain that increases the likelihood of depression might also be associated with a neuromuscular abnormality, which is presumably a factor contributing to the occurrence of OSA. Whether treatment with CPAP might affect these neurochemical alterations is unknown, but changes in some neurotransmitters or receptors have been observed.[9,13,23–30]

A patient who is depressed may experience an increase in sleep latency, a decrease in rapid eye movement (REM) latency, prolonged initial REM sleep, an increase in nighttime wakefulness, a decrease in slow-wave sleep (SWS), and early morning awakening.[31–33]

There is evidence for a link between depression and sleep-disordered breathing in the general population. It has been demonstrated that 800 out of 100,000 individuals have both a breathing-related sleep disorder and a major depressive disorder, with up to 20% of the subjects who presented with one of these disorders also having the other.[34,35]

Depression and OSA have each been shown to be associated independently with metabolic syndrome and also with the development of cardiovascular disease.[36–39] The association between depression and metabolic syndrome is thought to be reciprocal.[40] In particular, it has been suggested that a metabolic link exists between depressive disorder and atherosclerotic vascular diseases and insulin-resistance conditions.[41] Similarly, OSA has been observed to be independently associated with the cardiovascular risk factors comprising metabolic syndrome in particular, insulin resistance, and diabetes.[38,39]

The magnitude of this association has even led researchers to suggest that metabolic syndrome should encompass OSA.[42]

Possible Mechanisms Underlying the Association Between Depression and OSA: Shared Mechanisms

The 2 main factors suspected to be responsible for depressive symptoms in OSA are sleep fragmentation and oxygen desaturation during sleep. Sleep fragmentation is a direct consequence of the recurrent microarousals associated with the apneas and hypopneas, and the nocturnal hypoxemia is caused by the intermittent drops in oxygen saturation caused by the respiratory events.[43–45] Sleep fragmentation is the primary cause of EDS in patients with OSA, and is suggested to result in the symptoms of depression in OSA.[46,47] With respect to hypoxemia, it has been reported that the effect size of cognitive impairment in OSA is highly correlated with the severity of hypoxic events, ranging from 0.3 standard deviations for milder levels of the apnea hypopnea index (AHI) to 2 to 3 standard deviations for higher levels of AHI.[48]

In addition, preliminary imaging data suggest that hypoxemia related to OSA might also play a role in affecting mood.[43,48]

Neurobiology of Depression and Upper Airway Control in OSA: The Role of Serotonin

The high comorbidity of OSA and depression also suggests that both disorders may share a common neurobiological risk factor. On the neurotransmitter level, the serotoninergic system has a central role as a neurobiological substrate underlying impairments in the regulations of mood, sleep-wakefulness cycle, and upper airway muscle tone control during sleep. Depression is associated with a functional decrease of serotoninergic neurotransmission and is mostly responsible for the alterations in sleep as outlined earlier.[19,42,49–51]

The physiopathology of OSA involves numerous factors, among which the abnormal pharyngeal collapsibility during sleep is one of the most compelling. Serotonin (5-hydroxytryptamine; 5-HT) delivery to upper airway dilator motor neurons has been shown to be reduced in dependency of the vigilance state.[52] This reduction in 5-HT delivery leads to reductions in dilator muscle activity specifically during sleep, which may contribute to sleep apnea. Although the role of 5-HT in mood disorders has been largely documented, its involvement in the pathophysiology of sleep apnea remains to be understood. Molecules increasing the neurotransmission of the 5-HT, such as the selective serotonin reuptake inhibitors (SSRIs), are widely prescribed antidepressant molecules that are suggested to similarly improve the AHI in OSA. Serotoninergic drugs such as fluoxetine, protryptiline, and paroxetine have already been tested for OSA, with limited success and numerous adverse effects. Several 5-HT receptor ligands and bifunctional molecules are under development, which may be able to target both the depressive syndrome and OSA in the future.

MEDICATION-INDUCED APNEA

There are many medications that produce symptoms similar to those seen in OSA. Clinically this is of particular concern, because sedative antidepressants and adjunct treatments for depression may actually exacerbate OSA. Of note, hypnotics prescribed to treat depression-related insomnia might further decrease the muscle tone in the already functionally impaired upper airway dilator muscles, blunt the arousal response to hypoxia and hypercapnia, and increase the arousal threshold for the apneic event, thereby increasing the number and duration of apneas.[53,54]

These effects might differ depending on the patient population and the severity of OSA. Older depressive subjects are of primary concern; the frequencies of both OSA and depressive symptoms increase with age, as do prescription and consumption of sedative psychotropic medication. Pharmacologic treatment of depression and depression-related insomnia in this age group should therefore routinely consider the potential presence of a concomitant OSA.

Sedative antidepressants (eg, amitriptyline) and sedative neuroleptics (eg, chlorpromazine, clozapine) may impair performance and cause daytime drowsiness.

β-Blockers, especially lipophilic compounds (eg, metoprolol, propranolol), have been associated with difficulty in initiating sleep, an increased number of awakenings, and vivid dreams.

The chronic use of sedative-hypnotics often confounds normal sleep-wake functioning because of drug withdrawal effects or daytime drowsiness.[52,55]

The xanthines theophylline and caffeine are stimulants that increase wakefulness while they decrease SWS and total sleep time. The effect of caffeine can last as long as 8 to 14 hours, and may be more pronounced in older patients because of decreased caffeine clearance with decreased liver function. Furthermore, caffeine is present in many over-the-counter medications, including analgesics, cold or allergy remedies, appetite suppressants, and tonics used for fatigue, anorexia, and debility.

CLINICAL APPLICATION

There is a complex relationship between depression and OSA. It makes common sense for clinicians who treat either of these conditions to familiarize themselves with the signs and symptoms of both conditions. It might be beneficial for psychiatrists to consider obtaining a more comprehensive sleep history and familiarize themselves with a focused physical examination of the head and neck, including a simple oral examination to assess the tonsils, tongue, and uvula as well as the size and relative positions of their

patient's jaws. The mental health specialist should suspect OSA particularly in those depressed patients who present with compelling symptoms such as loud snoring or intermittent pauses in respiration as witnessed by a bed partner, associated with EDS. Other nocturnal symptoms may include restlessness, nocturia, excessive salivation and sweating, gastroesophageal reflux, as well as headache and dry mouth or throat in the morning on awakening.

When a patient is medically or surgically treated for OSA, the practitioner must realize that there could be an underlying psychological issue, and a referral to an appropriate mental health specialist must be considered. Conversely, an individual who is being treated for depression or other psychological issues and is resistant to treatment should also be evaluated for possible coexistence of OSA and referred to the appropriate specialist or team for further evaluation. The diagnosis and treatment of OSA might improve not only compliance with pharmacologic antidepressant treatment but also the treatment response rate for depression.[7,34,55-58]

SUMMARY

Sleep problems are more likely to affect patients with psychiatric disorders than people in the general population. Sleep problems may increase the risk for developing particular mental illnesses, and they may also arise as a result of such disorders. There is evidence to support the concept that treating sleep disorders may help to address psychological issues. The type of sleep disorder and its effect on mental health vary by psychiatric diagnosis. However, the overlap between disturbed sleep and psychological disorders is so great that researchers have long suspected that both types of problems may share common biologic roots.

Although the most common signs of OSA, including snoring, cessation of breathing while asleep, daytime somnolence, and restless sleep are well understood, the psychological issues may be more difficult to recognize and correctly diagnose. Humans require a certain amount of sleep to restore, repair, and recharge major organs down to the cellular level. These processes may not occur in patients with sleep apnea. The result is a patient who feels exhausted and drowsy in the morning and has an overpowering desire to sleep throughout the day. This condition produces frustration and irritability in patients because they must stay awake to perform their daily tasks. Problems with concentration and memory loss are also common. The impairments and associated emotions contribute to a growing sense of depression. Sufferers may even believe like they are losing their mind, because their ability to think clearly is diminished. The only desire may be to stay in bed and get the rest they think they need, when in reality they should be seeking treatment for their sleep disorder. In extreme cases, the psychological problems of sleep apnea may include thoughts of suicide. If the brain is continually deprived of oxygen night after night, the quality and purpose of a person's life steadily declines. Antidepressant drugs are not generally effective in these cases because the underlying sleep apnea must be diagnosed and effectively treated first.

Considering all that is known about sleep apnea and psychological disorders, it is highly advisable that patients who suffer from OSA be routinely evaluated with regard to the symptoms of depression. In addition, patients presenting primarily with symptoms of depression should be queried in an effort to uncover the possible presence of OSA. An analysis of these parameters may substantively affect the treatment of these patients.

Although researchers are still trying to understand all mechanisms involved, they have confirmed that sleep disruption—which affects the levels of neurotransmitters and stress hormones, among other things—wreaks havoc in the brain, impairing thinking and emotional regulation.

One final issue that is not addressed in this review is the psychological effect of untreated sleep apnea on the patient's bed partner. One can imagine that such correlation most certainly exists and, in many cases, may lead to marital dissatisfaction, spousal depression, agitation, and even divorce.

REFERENCES

1. Madani M, Madani F. Epidemiology, pathophysiology, and clinical features of obstructive sleep apnea. Oral Maxillofac Surg Clin North Am 2009;21:369–75.
2. Madani M, Madani F. The pandemic of obesity and its relationship to sleep apnea. Atlas Oral Maxillofac Surg Clin North Am 2007;15(2):81–8.
3. Ancoli-Israel S. Epidemiology of sleep disorders. Clin Geriatr Med 1989;5:347–62.
4. Madani M. Snoring and sleep apnea: a review article. Arch Iran Med 2007;10(2):215–26.
5. Guilleminault C, Stoohs R, Clerk A, et al. A cause of excessive daytime sleepiness. The upper airway resistance syndrome. Chest 1993;104:781–7.
6. Pillar G, Lavie P. Psychiatric symptoms in sleep apnea syndrome: effects of gender and respiratory disturbance index. Chest 1998;114:697–703.
7. Bardwell WA, Berry CC, Ancoli-Israel S, et al. Psychological correlates of sleep apnea. J Psychosom Res 1999;47:583–96.
8. Kales A, Caldwell AB, Cadieux RJ, et al. Severe obstructive sleep apnea—II: associated psychopathology and psychosocial consequences. J Chronic Dis 1985;38:427–34.
9. White J, Cates C, Wright J. Continuous positive airways pressure for obstructive sleep apnoea. Cochrane Database Syst Rev 2002;2:CD001106.
10. Derderian SS, Bridenbaugh RH, Rajagopal KR. Neuropsychologic symptoms in obstructive sleep apnea improve after treatment with nasal continuous positive airway pressure. Chest 1988;94:1023–7.
11. Engleman HM, Martin SE, Deary IJ, et al. Effect of continuous positive airway pressure treatment on daytime function in sleep apnoea/hypopnoea syndrome. Lancet 1994;343:572–5.
12. Engleman HM, Martin SE, Deary IJ, et al. Effect of CPAP therapy on daytime function in patients with mild sleep apnoea/hypopnoea syndrome. Thorax 1997;52:114–9.
13. Sanchez AI, Buela-Casal G, Bermudez MP, et al. The effects of continuous positive air pressure treatment on anxiety and depression levels in apnea patients. Psychiatry Clin Neurosci 2001;55:641–6.
14. McMahon JP, Foresman BH, Chisholm RC. The influence of CPAP on the neurobehavioral performance of patients with obstructive sleep apnea hypopnea syndrome: a systematic review. WMJ 2003;102:36–43.
15. Munoz A, Mayoralas LR, Barbe F, et al. Long-term effects of CPAP on daytime functioning in patients with sleep apnoea syndrome. Eur Respir J 2000;15:676–81.
16. Aikens JE, Vanable PA, Tadimeti L, et al. Differential rates of psychopathology symptoms in periodic limb movement disorder, obstructive sleep apnea, psychophysiological insomnia, and insomnia with psychiatric disorder. Sleep 1999;22:775–80.
17. Sforza E, de Saint Hilaire Z, Pelissolo A, et al. Personality, anxiety and mood traits in patients with sleep-related breathing disorders: effect of reduced daytime alertness. Sleep Med 2002;3:139–45.
18. Kaplan R. Obstructive sleep apnoea and depression—diagnostic and treatment implications. Aust N Z J Psychiatry 1992;26:586–91.
19. Aloia MS, Arnedt JT, Davis JD, et al. Neuropsychological sequelae of obstructive sleep apnea-hypopnea syndrome: a critical review. J Int Neuropsychol Soc 2004;10:772–85.
20. Li HY, Huang YS, Chen NH, et al. Mood improvement after surgery for obstructive sleep apnea. Laryngoscope 2004;114:1098–102.
21. Dahlof P, Ejnell H, Hallstrom T, et al. Surgical treatment of sleep apnea syndrome reduces associated major depression. Int J Behav Med 2000;7:73–88.

22. Andrews JG, Oei TP. The roles of depression and anxiety in the understanding and treatment of obstructive sleep apnea syndrome. Clin Psychol Rev 2004;24:1031–49.

23. D'Ambrosio C, Bowman T, Mohsenin V. Quality of life in patients with obstructive sleep apnea: effect of nasal continuous airway pressure; a prospective study. Chest 1999;115:123–9.

24. Means MK, Lichstein KL, Edinger JD, et al. Changes in depressive symptoms after continuous positive airway pressure treatment for obstructive sleep apnea. Sleep Breath 2003;7(1):31–42.

25. Ramos Platon MJ, Espinar Sierra J. Changes in psychopathological symptoms in sleep apnea patients after treatment with nasal continuous positive airway pressure. Int J Neurosci 1992;62:173–95.

26. Borak J, Cieslicki JK, Koziej M, et al. Effects of CPAP treatment on psychological status in patients with severe obstructive sleep apnoea. J Sleep Res 1996;5:123–7.

27. Yu BH, Ancoli-Israel S, Dimsdale JE. Effect of CPAP treatment on mood states in patients with sleep apnea. J Psychiatr Res 1999;33:427–32.

28. Henke KG, Grady JJ, Kuna ST. Effect of nasal continuous positive airway pressure on neuropsychological function in sleep apnea-hypopnea syndrome. A randomized, placebo-controlled trial. Am J Respir Crit Care Med 2001;163:911–7.

29. Millman RP, Fogel BS, McNamara ME, et al. Depression as a manifestation of obstructive sleep apnea: reversal with nasal continuous positive airway pressure. J Clin Psychiatry 1989;50:348–51.

30. Bardwell WA, Moore P, Ancoli-Israel S, et al. Fatigue in obstructive sleep apnea: driven by depressive symptoms instead of apnea severity? Am J Psychiatry 2003;160:350–5.

31. Baran AS, Richert AC. Obstructive sleep apnea and depression. CNS Spectr 2003;8:128–34.

32. Gregory AM, Rijsdijk FV, Lau JY, et al. The direction of longitudinal associations between sleep problems and depression symptoms: a study of twins aged 8 and 10 years. Sleep 2009;32(2):189–99.

33. Cho HJ, Lavretsky H, Olmstead R, et al. Sleep disturbance and depression recurrence in community-dwelling older adults: a prospective study. Am J Psychiatry 2008;165(12):1543–50.

34. Ohayon MM. The effects of breathing-related sleep disorders on mood disturbances in the general population. J Clin Psychiatry 2003;64:1195–200 [quiz: 1274–6].

35. Klonoff H, Fleetham J, Taylor DR, et al. Treatment outcome of obstructive sleep apnea: physiological and neuropsychological concomitants. J Nerv Ment Dis 1987;175:208–12.

36. Gami AS, Somers VK. Obstructive sleep apnoea, metabolic syndrome, and cardiovascular outcomes. Eur Heart J 2004;25:709–11.

37. Lett HS, Blumenthal JA, Babyak MA, et al. Depression as a risk factor for coronary artery disease: evidence, mechanisms, and treatment. Psychosom Med 2004;66:305–15.

38. Coughlin SR, Mawdsley L, Mugarza JA, et al. Obstructive sleep apnoea is independently associated with an increased prevalence of metabolic syndrome. Eur Heart J 2004;25:735–41.

39. Ip MS, Lam B, Ng MM, et al. Obstructive sleep apnea is independently associated with insulin resistance. Am J Respir Crit Care Med 2002;165:670–6.

40. Raikkonen K, Matthews KA, Kuller LH. The relationship between psychological risk attributes and the metabolic syndrome in healthy women: antecedent or consequence? Metabolism 2002;51:1573–7.

41. Ramasubbu R. Insulin resistance: a metabolic link between depressive disorder and atherosclerotic vascular diseases. Med Hypotheses 2002;59:537–51.

42. Wilcox I, McNamara SG, Collins FL, et al. "Syndrome Z": the interaction of sleep apnoea, vascular risk factors and heart disease. Thorax 1998;53(Suppl 3):S25–8.

43. Cohen-Zion M, Stepnowsky C, Marler, et al. Changes in cognitive function associated with sleep disordered breathing in older people. J Am Geriatr Soc 2001;49:1622–7.

44. Bardwell WA, Moore P, Ancoli-Israel S, et al. Does obstructive sleep apnea confound sleep architecture findings in subjects with depressive symptoms? Biol Psychiatry 2000;48:1001–9.

45. Reynolds CF, Kupfer DJ, McEachran AB, et al. Depressive psychopathology in male sleep apneics. J Clin Psychiatry 1984;45:287–90.

46. Vandeputte M, de Weerd A. Sleep disorders and depressive feelings: a global survey with the Beck Depression Scale. Sleep Med 2003;4:343–5.

47. Mosko S, Zetin M, Glen S, et al. Self-reported depressive symptomatology, mood ratings, and treatment outcome in sleep disorders patients. J Clin Psychol 1989;45:51–60.

48. Engleman HM, Kingshott RN, Martin SE, et al. Cognitive function in the sleep apnea/hypopnea syndrome (SAHS). Sleep 2000;23(Suppl 4):S102–8.

49. Adrien J. Neurobiological bases for the relation between sleep and depression. Sleep Med Rev 2002;6:341–51.

50. Germain A, Buysse DJ, Nofzinger E. Sleep-specific mechanisms underlying post-traumatic stress disorder: integrative review and neurobiological hypotheses. Sleep Med Rev 2008;12(3):185–95.

51. Shaffer J, Hoffman R, Armitage R. The neurobiology of depression: perspectives from animal and human sleep studies. Neuroscientist 2003;9:82–98.

52. Veasey SC. Serotonin agonists and antagonists in obstructive sleep apnea: therapeutic potential. Am J Respir Med 2003;2:21–9.

53. Miles LE, Dement WC. Sleep and aging. Sleep 1980; 3:1–220.

54. Guilleminault C. Benzodiazepines, breathing, and sleep. Am J Med 1990;88:25S–8S.

55. Farney RJ, Lugo A, Jensen RL, et al. Simultaneous use of antidepressant and antihypertensive medications increases likelihood of diagnosis of obstructive sleep apnea syndrome. Chest 2004; 125:1279–85.

56. Fleming JA, Fleetham JA, Taylor DR, et al. A case report of obstructive sleep apnea in a patient with bipolar affective disorder. Can J Psychiatry 1985;30:437–9.

57. Krystal AD. Sleep and psychiatric disorders: future directions. Psychiatr Clin North Am 2006;29(4):1115–30.

58. Akashiba T, Kawahara S, Akahoshi T, et al. Relationship between quality of life and mood or depression in patients with severe obstructive sleep apnea syndrome. Chest 2002;122:861–5.

Eating Disorders and the Oral and Maxillofacial Surgeon

Meredith Blitz, DDS[a,b,c,]*, David S. Rosen, MD, MPH[d,e,f,g]

KEYWORDS

- Eating disorders • Oral surgery • Electrolytes
- Complications

Perhaps the most challenging of all patients seeking treatment with the oral and maxillofacial surgeon (OMS) are those with eating disorders (EDs). Complex psychiatric illnesses, with their associated and significant medical sequelae, make a thorough knowledge of these disorders critical in the approach, evaluation, treatment planning, and surgical outcome in this expanding population of patients. Whether surgery for patients with EDs is elective in nature or unplanned, challenges are faced in all aspects of their care from diagnosis to preoperative preparation, surgery, and treatment. This article identifies and outlines issues of importance for the OMS when encountering patients with known or suspected EDs and provides guidance in the management of their outpatient or inpatient treatment.

DEFINITION, INCIDENCE AND EPIDEMIOLOGY

EDs are defined by the *Diagnostic and Statistical Manual of Mental Disorders, Fourth Edition-Text Revision* (DSM-IV-TR) and include any of several conditions characterized by serious disturbances of eating behavior. Most often considered are anorexia nervosa (AN) and bulimia nervosa (BN). Binge-eating disorder (BED) is a discrete entity listed only provisionally in the DSM-IV-TR but has been proposed for full inclusion in DSM-V.

AN is defined as a disorder characterized by a pathologic fear of gaining weight, leading to dysfunctional eating patterns, inadequate intake, severe malnutrition, and excessive weight loss (or in the case of growing adolescents, failure to gain weight appropriately). To reach the diagnostic threshold for AN, patients must meet 4 criteria. Refusal to maintain a body weight at or higher than the minimally expected weight for one's age and height is the primary criterion. Also included in diagnostic criteria are intense fear of becoming fat or gaining weight, disturbance in the way in which one's body is perceived, and in women who would be expected to be menstruating, amenorrhea (3 consecutive missed menstrual cycles). AN can be further categorized into restricting or binge/purge subtypes.

BN is a distinct eating disorder characterized by binge eating. Some compensatory behavior also

a Department of Oral and Maxillofacial Surgery, Division of Dentistry, Seton Hall University, 400 South Orange Avenue, South Orange, NJ 07079-2689, USA
b University of Medicine and Dentistry of New Jersey, 110 Bergen Street, Newark, NJ 07103, USA
c Department of Oral and Maxillofacial Surgery, St Joseph's Regional Medical Center, 703 Main Street, Paterson, NJ 07503, USA
d Department of Pediatrics and Communicable Disease, University of Michigan Medical School, Ann Arbor, MI, USA
e Department of Internal Medicine, University of Michigan Medical School, Ann Arbor, MI, USA
f Department of Psychiatry, University of Michigan Medical School, Ann Arbor, MI, USA
g Section of Teenage and Young Adult Health, Division of Child Behavioral Health, Department of Pediatrics, University of Michigan Health System, D3237 MPB Box 5718, 1500 East Medical Center Drive, Ann Arbor, MI 48109-5718, USA
* Corresponding author. Department of Oral and Maxillofacial Surgery, St Joseph's Regional Medical Center, 703 Main Street, Paterson, NJ 07503.
E-mail address: blitzgme@umdnj.edu

Oral Maxillofacial Surg Clin N Am 22 (2010) 511–517
doi:10.1016/j.coms.2010.07.008
1042-3699/10/$ — see front matter © 2010 Published by Elsevier Inc.

occurs aimed at "undoing" the binge, most commonly manual or pharmacologic self-induced vomiting but possibly laxative abuse or compulsive exercise. Feelings of guilt, shame, and depression can accompany the episodes. The primary criterion for BN diagnosis is recurrent episodes of binge eating when, in a discrete period of time, the patient eats a larger volume of food than most other people would eat in the same time period and experiences a loss of control over the episode. Compensatory behavior to prevent weight gain (eg, vomiting, laxatives, compulsive exercise) must be present to meet the criterion. The episodes occur at least twice a week for a period of 3 months, and there is excessive self-evaluation based on body shape/weight. Like AN, there are 2 subtypes: purging and nonpurging.

Estimates suggest that 0.5% of the population of adolescent girls in the United States have AN. Approximately 1% to 2% of adolescent girls meet the criteria for BN. The male sex accounts for 5% to 10% of all cases of disordered eating. According to data posted by the National Eating Disorders Association, AN and BN affects 10 million of the female sex and 1 million of the male and millions more suffer from BED. Patients who do not meet the strict criteria in the DSM IV manual for AN and BN are considered to have "partial syndromes" or "eating disorder − not otherwise specified" (ED-NOS). The prevalence of ED-NOS has been estimated to be as high as 14%. These patients may suffer from the same psychological and physiologic sequelae as those who do meet the strict criteria for AN and BN and may therefore pose precisely the same management challenges to the OMS.

The typical patient with an ED was previously thought to be an affluent, white, overachieving, thin, adolescent girl. Individuals, such as gymnasts, ballet dancers, and models, driven to maintain a lean body habitus for athletics or employment have also been recognized to be at significantly increased risk of developing EDs. However, EDs have been recently increasing amongst the male sex, minority populations, and in progressively younger patients. Forty percent of 9- and 10-year-old girls are trying to lose weight,[1] and a recent analysis from 1999 to 2006 revealed that hospitalizations for EDs rose most precipitously in children younger than 12 years.[2] Thus, the possibility of an ED in a patient with characteristic signs and symptoms must be considered regardless of age, gender, socioeconomic status, or ethnicity.

The cause of EDs is considered to be multifactorial. A strong genetic basis has been shown in family and twin studies.[3] Predisposition to certain traits, such as behavioral rigidity and perfectionism, which may be genetically determined, seems to contribute as well. The genetic component seems to be induced at puberty.[4,5] Like many neuropsychiatric illnesses, environmental interactions appear to play a role.[6] Dieting is also an important risk factor and several studies have shown that chronic repetitive dieting plays a significant proximal role in the development of EDs.[7−9] Gastrointestinal (GI) complaints may also precede EDs and should be considered as potential risk factors. Pediatric autoimmune neuropsychiatric disorder associated with streptococcus is a controversial syndrome that some believe may cause or contribute to AN in the adolescent and child population.

Unfortunately, even when considering the strong genetic component and concordance between twins, EDs are often not considered biologically based illnesses. This can limit access to care and insurance coverage, which makes successful diagnosis and treatment a health care challenge. Diagnosis is often delayed or sometimes even denied by the patient. Thus, a characteristic presentation and/or physical findings should alert the practitioner to the possibility of an ED even in the absence of a prior diagnosis.

ORGAN SYSTEM PATHOPHYSIOLOGY

EDs may affect each and every organ system. Medical complications can require hospitalization and can even be life-threatening. A comprehensive patient history of the disorder that covers onset, specific symptoms, and current level of disability is critical in the management of these patients before treatment. A standard approach to comprehensive evaluation is recommended.

Medical complications are common; fortunately, most resolve with successful treatment that includes refeeding and elimination of purging behaviors. Malnutrition is at the heart of many of the medical complications in AN and, early on, the body adapts. However, over time, the body's ability to compensate for inadequate nutritional intake leads to increasing symptoms related to energy deficits and consequent metabolic changes. Basal metabolism decreases, body temperature decreases, and organ systems are increasingly affected. Although most organ systems can recover with nutritional rehabilitation, statural growth deficits, structural brain alterations, and decreased bone mineral density may be irreversible.[10]

Cardiovascular organ system perturbations are considerable. Orthostatic blood pressure changes (with or without pulse changes), bradycardia, poor peripheral perfusion, and potentially, acrocyanosis can be seen. Repolarization abnormalities are potentially dangerous and should be referred for urgent evaluation. Pericardial effusions, functional mitral valve prolapse with murmur, myocardial muscle dysfunction, and ipecac-related cardiomyopathy are also possible.

Anemia is not uncommon, which can further exacerbate cardiac stress. Thrombocytopenia and immune suppression due to leukopenia have also been documented.

GI issues are common. GI complaints may precede the onset of an ED. Patients with EDs frequently have delayed gastric emptying time and increased intestinal transit time, which lead to a sense of fullness and bloating that can compromise successful refeeding and recovery. For patients with a history of vomiting, gastroesophageal reflux disease (GERD) is common. Mallory-Weiss tears are uncommon but catastrophic events. Constipation is extremely common and may be difficult to treat.

Endocrine abnormalities can be severe and are also common in the ED population. Hypothyroidism, hypercortisolism, hypogonadotropic hypogonadism, and euthyroid-sick syndrome (low free thyroxine, normal thyroid stimulating hormone) have all been identified in this population. Euthyroid-sick syndrome is common and does not require supplemental thyroid replacement hormone. Activation of the hypothalamic-pituitary-adrenal (HPA) axis contributes to appetite suppression and physical hyperactivity.[11] Hypothalamic suppression causes amenorrhea. Amenorrhea is an important marker for low bone density and its association with cognitive impairment in AN has also been suggested.[12] Growth retardation leading to short stature and pubertal delay may be seen in prepubertal and peripubertal individuals. The endocrine abnormalities causing failure of normal growth patterns include altered thyroid and adrenal function, decreased levels of the sex hormones, and uncoupling of growth hormone from insulinlike growth factor. Growth may never reach normal levels, because permanent effects on growth can occur.

The integumentary and musculoskeletal systems are likely to be affected and may provide some additional clinical findings to support the diagnosis of an ED. Skin changes often include lanugo hair, which is the return of the soft, downy hair that often covers a newborn child. Patients with an ED also have dry skin that may appear scaly or yellow, particularly on the palms and soles, characteristic of carotenemia. Attention should be given to the knuckles to determine the presence of Russell sign (calluses due to self-induced vomiting). Hair thinning and hair loss can occur and nail changes are also common.

Low bone mineral density is a frequent complication in both male and female patients. The patients are thus susceptible to increased risk of pathologic fractures, and, more importantly, this bone loss may be irreversible. Such compromise to the skeletal system can lead to lifelong difficulties.

The pathophysiology of the skeletal compromise is not limited to decreased intake of oral calcium and vitamin D. Other contributing factors include deficiency of the gonadal steroids, lack of muscle mass that leads to loss of mechanical stimulation of bone turnover and growth, and increase in cortisol levels by the activation of the HPA axis. Apart from nutritional and psychological rehabilitation, there is no proven therapy to reverse low bone mineral density. Supplemental calcium and vitamin D should be prescribed. However, neither supplemental hormonal therapy nor bisphosphonates have been shown to be effective enough to support their routine use. Any of these treatments, however, may have been previously attempted; therefore, oral health care providers should ask this patient population about bisphosphonate therapy to better recognize the increased risk of bisphosphonate-related osteonecrosis of the jaw.

Perhaps the most complex organ system changes occur in the brain. Gray and white matter deficits with associated increases in cerebrospinal fluid are proportional to weight loss in these patients. HPA axis dysfunction may lead to brain changes that are associated with elevated cortisol levels. The patient's affect may appear to be flat or anxious. Cognitive impairments are well-known in this population, and functional brain imaging studies have shown decreases in global and localized activity.[13] It is not known to what extent these changes are reversible. White matter volume changes seem to resolve with refeeding, whereas gray matter changes may persist despite increasing weight.[12,14]

LABORATORY VALUES

Abnormal serum electrolyte levels can compromise the ability of the OMS to perform procedures and administer anesthesia. Early on in the disease process, electrolytes may remain within normal range; however, hypokalemia, hypomagnesemia, hyponatremia, hypocalcemia, hypochloremic metabolic alkalosis (vomiting), and hyperchloremic metabolic acidosis (laxative abuse) have all been documented.

Hypokalemia is most often encountered in bulimic patients because of chronic vomiting and/or laxative abuse. Hypokalemia in a patient with an ED is often associated with protracted, frequent, or daily purging. Serum potassium levels of less than 3.2 mmol/L may require hospital admission. Patients with restrictive-type AN are less at risk of hypokalemia even in the presence of low weight.[15] Hypochloremia due to vomiting can occur and hospitalization may be required because of low serum chloride levels (<88 mmol/L). Hypochloremia may occur in up to 25% of patients.

Hypomagnesemia is also of concern. The incidence of hypomagnesemia has been reported to be as high as 25%.[16] Symptoms reported in this study included muscular weakness, cramping of the extremities, restlessness, paresthesias, diminished concentration, cardiac arrhythmias, hypertension, and diminished recent memory. The study did not consider concurrent hypocalcemia, which can occur in patients with low serum magnesium levels. Oral replacement therapy may reverse the symptoms associated with low magnesium levels. Hypocalcemia is rare and generally encountered only in the most severely affected patients.

Decreased serum sodium levels can be seen in patients who practice "water loading," that is ingesting large amounts of water in an attempt to feel "full" or to misrepresent their weight at medical visits. However, water intoxication is a significant danger and can lead to cerebral swelling, seizures, coma, and death. Dangerously low serum sodium levels have been reported. For patients who will require fluid therapy for outpatient anesthesia, it may be best to avoid intravenous (IV) solutions with substantial free water (eg, dextrose 5% in water) to prevent the potential complications of hyponatremia.

ORAL SURGERY CONCERNS/FINDINGS

OMSs, general practitioners, pediatric dentists, and orthodontists should be knowledgeable about EDs, because they may be the first health professionals to suspect them. Abnormalities of the hard and soft dental tissues are well-documented and should be easily detected by the oral health care provider. Female practitioners and dental hygienists may be more clinically astute to note oral findings related to EDs.[17,18]

Findings are many and include xerostomia (medication-induced, dehydration), caries (cervical level due to xerostomia), attrition, erosion (palatal surface of anterior teeth common), mucositis, loss of tongue papillae,[19] cheilosis (from vomiting and vitamin deficiencies), parotid hypertrophy (associated with hyperamylasemia), minor salivary gland sialadenosis,[20] necrotizing sialometaplasia,[21] and temporomandibular myofascial pain dysfunction.[22,23] Considering that the typical age at onset for EDs coincides with the need for evaluation and management of third molars, OMSs are in a position to note these findings and should maintain a high index of suspicion.

Xerostomia is a potential side effect of many of the medications sometimes prescribed for patients with EDs. Although none are currently Food and Drug Administration-approved for the primary treatment of AN, medications are often prescribed to treat comorbid anxiety or depression. Estimates of comorbidity between 40% and 60% have been suggested. Several pharmacologic agents have been shown to be effective in the management of BN. The most common class of medications used in patients with EDs is the selective serotonin reuptake inhibitors.

Dry mouth may be exacerbated in patients with dehydration and also may potentially contribute to decreased oral intake. To date, no studies have been undertaken to evaluate the role of xerostomia in progression of the disease process in patients with EDs.

Along with xerostomia, mucositis is common. Mucositis is defined as painful inflammation and ulceration of the digestive tract. Mucositis is extremely painful and oral intake is limited secondarily to pain. Mucositis can develop in the patient with dehydration and chronic exposure to stomach acid. The ulcerations can become secondarily infected leading to further complications. Loss of fungiform papillae of the tongue is another manifestation of oral mucosal change, however, this change was more commonly seen in patients with restrictive-type ED than in patients who vomited.[19]

Angular cheilosis is an inflammatory lesion found at the labial commissures, bilaterally producing deep cracks in the tissue. If the condition is severe enough, bleeding may occur with movement. Incrustations and ulcerations may also be found. Studies have linked the initial onset of angular cheilosis with nutritional deficiencies, specifically, riboflavin (vitamin B2) and zinc deficiency and iron deficiency anemia. These causes may indicate a poor diet and malnutrition. Should they be superinfected with candidal species or bacteria, medical management is advised. Lesions should resolve with refeeding, and with improved nutritional status if malnutrition is the primary cause.

Multiple salivary gland lesions and alterations have been noted in patients with EDs. Parotid hypertrophy is the most well-known of the salivary changes; however, minor salivary gland sialadenosis is common as well, and necrotizing sialometaplasia has been documented.

Painless bilateral swelling of the parotid, submandibular, or other salivary glands is frequently found in patients who vomit/purge. The incidence of parotid gland swelling has been reported in up to 15% of BN patients. The pathogenesis is unknown, but it has been suggested to involve an autonomic neuropathy associated with frequent emesis. With impairment of the sympathetic nervous system, acinar cells within the gland enlarge because of zymogen granule engorgement.[24] Zymogen is the precursor of amylase, and parotid hypertrophy has been associated with hyperamylasemia. Because amylase levels are salivary rather than pancreatic, vomiting, not binging, is most probably responsible for the elevation.[25]

Oral complications are not only limited to the soft-tissue structures. Dental erosion, attrition, and caries are common and lead to an overall deterioration in the patient's aesthetics, ability to masticate, and, ultimately, quality of life. Erosion of the enamel surfaces of the teeth is common in the ED patient with chronic vomiting. Excessive exposure to stomach acids leads to the classic pattern of erosion of the palatal surfaces of the anterior maxillary teeth. Erosion can be seen on all surfaces and the practitioner should note all involved areas on examination. As mentioned previously, caries at the cervical level is due to decreased salivary flow and may require advanced dental procedures.

Attrition of the occlusal surfaces of the teeth indicates excessive wear. Women with EDs, specifically vomiting, have been found to have higher sensitivity to muscle palpation than nonvomiting patients. They have also been found to sometimes have intensive gum chewing, ice chewing, or other compulsive oral habits that may contribute to myofascial pain.[22] Research has also shown that patients with ED are more likely to suffer from chronic facial pain. Using a digital analog scale, more than 60% of patients reported current or previous facial pain.[23]

RISK OF RELAPSE

For the OMS and other dental surgical subspecialists, the greatest postoperative concern is the risk of ED relapse. This area has not been extensively studied. Considering the age range during which most patients seek third molar extraction surgery and its close relationship to the high-risk age range

for EDs, it might be beneficial to explore the issue of relapse.

In 2001, Maine and Goldberg[26] investigated the role of dental surgery in the etiology and course of EDs. The methodology involved questions included in a pretreatment assessment for new patients entering an ED therapy program during a 22-month period. The questions were designed to obtain information regarding the effects of oral procedures on the patients' EDs.

The study revealed that dental procedures significantly altered the course of the patient's ED. Third molar surgery was specifically listed as a risk factor for exacerbation and relapse. No respondents reported that dental procedures were the causative factor in the initial development of their ED. However, 9.3% of respondents indicated that dental treatment had caused exacerbation or relapse. Of most concern was that 38% of patients who responded in the affirmative to exacerbation due to dental treatment indicated that third molar surgery was a causative factor.[26]

Three case reports published in 2007 also postulate a possible role of dental treatment in precipitating weight loss leading to AN.[27] The potential role of dental and oral surgical treatment in the initiation and relapse of ED requires further examination and research.

Any patient with a history of an ED should be assessed and managed by a health care team that includes a pediatrician, a family physician or general internal medicine physician, a registered dietician, and a mental health professional. Collateral information from family members may be helpful in assessing risk. Consultation with an anesthesiologist should be considered if general anesthesia may be required. In any patient who is actively symptomatic or for whom remission from their ED is incomplete or uncertain, delaying surgery until the patient is more clinically stable should be considered. All elective oral surgical procedures should be delayed until an adequate assessment of the current physical status of the patient has been completed. In the case of emergent surgery, hospitalization may be indicated for monitoring of patient fluids and electrolytes, intravenous medication delivery, nutritional interventions, and pain management and to ensure access to the comprehensive resources needed for management during the pre- and postoperative periods (**Box 1**).

Patients who undergo third molar surgery or other oral surgical procedures should be counseled extensively about the effects of dehydration and malnutrition on healing. Delayed wound healing can lead to extended periods of pain and limited oral intake. Assurance of adequate

Box 1
Management of patients with ED

1. Thorough current history from the patient and family
   - must include medication use, substance abuse history, disease activity
2. Consultation with the ED treatment team
3. Laboratory values
   - Complete blood count with differential
   - Chemistry profile with electrolytes
   - Serum magnesium level
   - Liver function tests
   - Coagulation profile
   - Urinalysis
4. Electrocardiogram
5. Anesthesia consultation
6. Mental health consultation (pre- and postoperative)
7. Nutritional counseling for postoperative dietary management

Box 2
Potential oral surgical complications in patients with EDs

1. Relapse/exacerbation of disordered eating
2. Acute weight loss
3. Dehydration
4. Bleeding
5. Infection
6. Delayed wound healing
7. Anxiety related to physical changes and appearance
8. Fluid overload (with IV fluids)
9. Medication interactions

nutritional intake should be one of the primary steps when the surgical intervention is considered. This should be discussed with all patients, their families, and their treatment teams before elective surgery.

The anesthetic risk is considerable for affected patients. Medical consultation should be sought to assess the suitability of the patient for sedation or general anesthesia. The risk of complications related to electrolyte disturbances, fluid imbalances, dehydration, substance abuse, GERD, delayed GI transport, anemia, thrombocytopenia, and concomitant medication usage is significant. Poor peripheral perfusion may affect the accuracy of usual monitoring devices (eg, pulse oximetry) in ED patients. Hospitalization for nonemergent and elective cases should be considered to avoid catastrophic events and to allow for multiple practitioners to have access to the patient during the presurgical, surgical, and postoperative phases of care.

If the patient is to receive care in the outpatient setting because of health insurance limitations or minimal level of surgical difficulty, laboratory values should be current and corrected before care. Patients are best managed with local anesthesia with or without nitrous oxide analgesia. Medically stable patients may benefit from appropriately titrated moderate sedation.. For the patient who presents for consultation for surgery with any clinical signs or symptoms of an ED but denies such a history, the practitioner should avoid all elective surgery until further information can be gathered (**Box 2**).

SUMMARY

Individuals with ED are among the most challenging patients treated by the OMS. There are many issues that must be considered before elective and emergent care. For the OMS and other dental practitioners, particularly those who treat adolescents, it is critical to have a solid understanding of the pathophysiology and the potential complications of ED. Management of patients with EDs requires a team approach to care, and early consultation with the patient's treatment team is indicated when oral surgical procedures are anticipated. This is critically important considering the role that oral care may have on the initiation and relapse of these diseases.

REFERENCES

1. Schreiber GB, Robins M, Striegel-Moore R, et al. Weight modification efforts reported by black and white preadolescent girls: national heart, lung, and blood institute growth and health study. Pediatrics 1996;98(1):63–70.
2. Agency for Healthcare and Quality Research. Eating disorders sending more Americans to the hospital. AHRQ news and numbers. Rockville (MD): U.S. Department of Health and Human services; 2009.
3. Strober M, Freeman R, Lampert C, et al. Controlled family study of anorexia nervosa and bulimia nervosa: evidence of shared liability and transmission of partial syndromes. Am J Psychiatry 2000;157: 393–401.
4. Klump KL, McGue M, Iacono WG. Differential heritability of eating attitudes and behaviors in prepubertal versus pubertal twins. Int J Eat Disord 2003; 33:287–92.
5. Klump K, Gobrogge KL, Perkins PS, et al. Preliminary evidence that gonadal hormones organize and activate disordered eating. Psychol Med 2006; 36:539–46.

6. Mazzeo SE, Bulik CM. Environmental and genetic risk factors for eating disorders: what the clinician needs to know. Child Adolesc Psychiatr Clin N Am 2008;18:67–82.

7. Streigel-Moore RH, Bulik CM. Risk factors for eating disorders. Am Psychol 2007;62:181–98.

8. McKnight Investigators. Risk factors for the onset of eating disorders in adolescent girls: results of the McKnight longitudinal risk factor study. Am J Psychiatry 2003;160:248–54.

9. Neumark-Sztainer D, Wall M, Guo J, et al. Obesity, disordered eating, and eating disorders in a longitudinal study of adolescents: how do dieters fare 5 years later? J Am Diet Assoc 2006;106:559–68.

10. Katzman DK. Medical complications in adolescents with anorexia nervosa: a review of the literature. Int J Eat Disord 2005;37:S52–9.

11. Sauro CL, Ravaldi C, Cabras PL, et al. Stress, hypothalamic-pituitary-adrenal axis and eating disorders. Neuropsychobiology 2008;57:95–115.

12. Chui HT, Christensen BK, Zipursky RB, et al. Cognitive function and brain structure in females with a history of adolescent-onset anorexia nervosa. Pediatrics 2008;122:e426–37.

13. Van den Eynde F, Treasure J. Neuroimaging in eating disorders and obesity: implications for research. Child Adolesc Psychiatr Clin N Am 2008; 18:95–115.

14. Katzman DK, Zipursky RB, Lambe EK, et al. Longitudinal magnetic resonance imaging study of the brain changes in adolescents with anorexia nervosa. Arch Pediatr Adolesc Med 1997;151:793–7.

15. Greenfeld D, Mickley D, Quinlan DM, et al. Hypokalemia in outpatients with eating disorders. Am J Psychiatry 1995;152:60–3.

16. Hall R, Hoffman R, Beresford T, et al. Hypomagnesemia in patients with eating disorders. Psychosomatics 1988;29:264–72.

17. Bretz WA. Oral indicators of eating disorders are more readily detected by female than male dentists. J Evid Based Dent Pract 2007;7(2):86–7.

18. Debate RD, Vogel E, Tedesco LA, et al. Sex differences among dentists regarding eating disorders and secondary prevention practices. J Am Dent Assoc 2006;137(6):773–81.

19. Wockel L, Jacob A, Holtmann M, et al. Reduced number of taste papillae in patients with eating disorders. J Neural Transm 2009;115(3):537–44.

20. Aframian DJ. Anorexia/bulimia-related sialadenosis of palatal minor salivary glands. J Oral Pathol Med 2005;34(6):383.

21. Solomon LW, Merzianu M, Sullivan M, et al. Necrotizing sialometaplasia associated with bulimia: case report and literature review. Oral Surg Oral Med Oral Pahol Oral Radiol Endod 2007;103(2):e39–42.

22. Emodi-Perlman A, Yoffe T, Rosenberg N, et al. Prevalence of psychologic, dental and temporomandibular signs and symptoms among chronic eating disorders patients: a comparative control study. J Orofac Pain 2008;22(3):201–8.

23. Goldberg MB, Katzman DK, Woodside DB, et al. Do eating disorders and chronic facial pain coexist? A preliminary study. J Can Dent Assoc 2006;72(1):51.

24. Mandel L, Abai S. Diagnosing bulimia nervosa with parotid gland swelling. J Am Dent Assoc 2004;135(5):613–6.

25. Robertson C, Millar H. Hyperamylasemia in bulimia nervosa and hyperemesis gravidarum. Int J Eat Disord 1999;26(2):223–7.

26. Maine M, Goldberg M. The role of third molar surgery in the exacerbation of eating disorders. J Oral Maxillofac Surg 2001;59:1297–300.

27. Jaffa T. Three cases illustrating the potential of dental treatment as a precipitant for weight loss leading to anorexia nervosa. Eur Eat Disord Rev 2007;15(1):42–4.

End-of-Life Issues for the Oral and Maxillofacial Surgeon

Renie Daniel, DMD, MS[a],*, John J. Mitchell Jr, PhD[b],
Paul E. Gates, DDS, MBA[c,d]

KEYWORDS

- End-of-life • Ethical principles
- Oral and maxillofacial surgery • Cancer

During a career of clinical practice, the oral and maxillofacial surgeon (OMS) encounters a host of challenges. These challenges require excellence in clinical competence and a keen awareness of the ethical dimensions of patient care. There are times when the ethical dimensions of clinical practice must be the primary focus. A commitment to these ethical dimensions has always been an important part of the practice of oral and maxillofacial surgery, and this remains true today.[1] However, developments in medicine and society in the course of the last several decades have increased the responsibility of physicians to be attentive to the ethical values at the core of the patient-physician relationship. This heightened ethical responsibility applies to every dimension of the OMS's clinical practice, especially when engaged in the care of a terminally ill patient.[2] Although other physicians may share a measure of responsibility for the care of the patient, for example, an oncologist who has treated a patient with head or neck cancer, the OMS who has treated the patient in the earlier stages of his illness retains a responsibility to the patient until the end.[3] How this responsibility is exercised may make a difference in whether the dignity of the patient is protected and nourished in the last months,

weeks, and days of life. When the curative stage of patient care has been exhausted because no more treatments are available to reverse or slow the progress of a terminal disease, the palliative stage of care emerges as the top priority in the physician-patient relationship. Although other clinicians may also be engaged in this dimension of patient care, the OMS would often have some unique contributions to the patient's care and comfort.[4] The OMS should maintain the relationship with the patient that has developed over years and months. The continuity of this relationship often brings a special comfort as death draws near to patient and family.

This discussion of the responsibilities of the OMS in providing end-of-life care is presented in two parts. Part I examines the ethical values that should shape the OMS's care of the terminally ill patient. Attention is also focused on how the evolving nature of the physician-patient relationship shapes the dynamics of providing patient care at the end of life. Part II examines the specific clinical aspects of the OMS's care of the terminally ill patient in the provision of end-of-life care. Particularly significant is the shift in focus of the physician-patient relationship when the primary emphasis becomes preserving the comfort and

The authors have nothing to disclose.
[a] Department of Oral and Maxillofacial Surgery, St Joseph's Regional Medical Center, 703 Main Street, Paterson, NJ 07503, USA
[b] Department of Biomedical Ethics, School of Health and Medical Sciences, Seton Hall University, 400 South Orange Avenue, South Orange, NJ 07079, USA
[c] Department of Dentistry, Bronx Lebanon Hospital Center, 1770 Grand Concourse, Bronx, NY 10457, USA
[d] Department of Dentistry, Dr Martin Luther King Community Health Center, 1650 Grand Concourse, Bronx, NY 10457, USA
* Corresponding author.
E-mail address: rdaniel529@gmail.com

dignity of the patient after medicine's curative options have been exhausted.

PART I

During the last several decades, many significant changes have occurred in American culture and society, perhaps none more dramatic than those in the nature of the patient-physician relationship. The paternalistic assumptions that had shaped the relationship between physicians and patients for centuries and gave physicians almost exclusive authority in medical decision-making have given way to a partnership enabling patients to exercise a more significant role in decisions about their medical care.[5] In a special way, this shift has been manifested in the right of patients to more fully participate in decisions about their care at the end of life. Although these changes have not come without a struggle, today, physicians and patients alike recognize and accept the need for a shared decision-making model. Patients make decisions about their medical care based on their values and goals. The changing nature of the physician-patient relationship challenges the OMS to adjust to a new formula about how decisions are made in patient care, especially when caring for terminally ill and dying patients. Recent research indicates that patients with terminal illnesses and those whose lives are otherwise at risk want to be fully informed about the reasonable choices available, so that decisions appropriate to each individual's care can be made.[6] Just 40 years ago, research indicated that a significant majority of oncologists caring for terminally ill patients decided how much patients should be told about their diagnosis and prognosis.[7] Today, telling the truth and transparency have become the ethical standard in communications between physicians and patients with serious illnesses. This standard is embodied in the codes of ethics of professional medical societies.[8]

In the effort to provide excellence in patient care at the end of life, several positive developments can be identified. These developments support the OMS's commitment to patient-centered care at the outset of the twenty-first century. The ethical principles and values central to providing end-of-life care have been articulated clearly and forcefully. Furthermore, during the last several decades, millions of dollars have been invested in the education of physicians in the competencies required for providing patient-centered end-of-life care. Hospitals and other health care institutions have embraced the goal of excellence in end-of-life care, providing physicians with various forms of support to attain this goal, including

ethics committees that can provide a consultation service when physicians confront especially challenging ethical dilemmas. The growth of palliative care medicine and the hospice movement can assist the OMS in the transition from the curative to the palliative stage of patient care. The enactment of advance directives statutes in all 50 states enables patients to articulate their wishes about medical care at the end of life, with the expectation that their wishes will be respected even when they are unable to participate in the medical decision-making process. Finally, the jurisprudence regarding the rights of patients at the end of life has been clarified.[9] Patients have the right to make decisions consistent with their values and goals. These positive developments offer a framework supporting the OMS's efforts to place the terminally ill patient at the center of medical decision-making.

Despite these positive developments in support of the OMS's efforts to advance excellence in end-of-life care, obstacles remain. The United States remains a predominantly death-denying culture. It is impossible to determine whether this is the result of secularization or simply a fear of dying. Physicians frequently confront a challenge when terminally ill patients or their family members deny the inevitability of death. The history of medical practice embodies a paradigm in which death is viewed as the enemy to be defeated at all costs, and for many physicians, the patient's death is viewed as a personal failure. The OMS faces the challenge of supporting the dying patient without harboring feelings of personal failure. Recent studies indicate that many physicians remain mesmerized by potentially life-prolonging technologies. Imposing such interventions on unwilling patients violates their right of self-determination. The quality of the physician's communication with the terminally ill patient is, at times, inadequate. Only informed patients can make informed decisions. OMSs should be committed to transparency so that their patients can make decisions consistent with the medical facts and their values and goals. Finally, a lack of cultural competence can impede the delivery of patient-centered end-of-life care. OMSs who care for diverse patient populations should be aware of and sensitive to how patients from different ethnic, cultural, racial, and religious groups diverge in their understanding of the process of dying.

The ethical framework for providing patients with the end-of-life care consistent with their values, goals, and wishes can be found in the ethical principles that should shape and guide the OMS. The principle of beneficence imposes on the OMS the obligation to seek the good of the patient in accordance with the wishes of the patient. In end-of-life care, beneficence establishes a responsibility to ascertain the goals of the patient and to act in manner consistent with these goals. The principle of nonmalfeasance imposes an ethical obligation to refrain from intentionally harming the patient, that is, above all, "do no harm." In end-of-life care, this principle establishes an obligation to neither harm by omission (a failure to treat) nor by commission (providing unwanted or nonbeneficial treatments). The principle of autonomy, the centerpiece of the change that has occurred in the nature of the patient-physician relationship, refers to the potential of the individual to be self-determining. In end-of-life care, autonomy defines the right of patients to decide on the best course of treatment or no treatment in consultation with their physician and to have these wishes respected. The principle of veracity pertains to the OMS's obligation to tell patients the truth about their medical condition. In end-of-life care, knowing the truth, as best as it can be known, is the foundation on which patients make decisions about how they wish to be cared for in the last months and weeks of their lives. The principle of fidelity pertains to the OMS's responsibility to be an advocate for the patient. In end-of-life care, fidelity pertains to the obligation to support the lawful wishes of the patient, even when these wishes may differ from the preferences of the physician. The principle of proportionate versus disproportionate means pertains to the process by which a patient weighs the benefits and burdens of various courses of treatment or of no treatment. The principle asks: (1) What is the usefulness of the treatment? (2) What are the benefits and burdens of various possible courses of treatment or no treatment? (3) How do patients, in accordance with their values and goals, weigh the benefits and burdens of the various possible treatments or of no treatment? and (4) What course of treatment does the patient wish to pursue or does the patient wish for no treatment? The challenge for the OMS is to assist the patient in understanding and then evaluating the various possible courses of treatment in accordance with the wishes, values, and goals of the patient for end-of-life care.

As a new ethical framework for decision-making at the end of life has evolved during the last several decades, a parallel development has defined the legal right of patients to fully participate in the decision-making process. This development has come as a comfort to patients, family members, and physicians. The legal rights of patients have been articulated in state and federal statutes and case law. At the center of these legal rights is an unequivocal defense of the declaration that the primary focus of end-of-life care must be the wishes of the patient. Authority in the decision-making process has shifted from the physician or other caregiver to the patient. Today, the OMS understands that a patient's constitutionally protected right to privacy includes the right to refuse any and all medical treatments and interventions, including potentially life-prolonging medical interventions. The patient's right to self-determination is not diminished when the patient is no longer able to participate in the medical decision-making process. The prior expressed wishes of the patient retain the authority to direct the appropriate course of treatment and should not be set aside. Family members or other surrogates who act on behalf of the patient who is no longer able to participate in the decision-making process should be guided in their decisions by the known wishes and values of the patient. The law has firmly established that neither brain death nor the diagnosis of a persistent vegetative state are a necessary precondition for withholding or withdrawing potentially life-prolonging medical interventions. Patients have a constitutional right to refuse any and all medical interventions that are judged to be contrary to their wishes and values. Furthermore, life-prolonging medical interventions include treatments as simple as antibiotics to the use of mechanical ventilation. It is well-established that there is neither an ethical nor a legal distinction between a decision to withhold a potentially life-prolonging medical intervention and a decision to withdraw such an intervention. The wishes of the patient should prevail in either circumstance. Finally, the jurisprudence that has evolved with respect to the patient's right to decide about end-of-life care eliminates the need to subject these decisions to judicial review. A fundamental goal of this jurisprudence has been to protect the integrity of the patient-physician relationship without undue interference from third parties. Patients in consultation with their physician are the centerpiece of the decision-making process in matters pertaining to end-of-life care.

The social, ethical, and legal developments that have clarified the authority of the patient and the nature of the patient-physician relationship can fortify the OMS in a commitment to providing excellence in end-of-life care for patients. This dimension of patient care fortunately does not dominate the OMS's clinical practice. However, when called upon to support a terminally ill or dying patient, the OMS has no greater moral responsibility. When the nature of the relationship with the patient transitions from the curative to the palliative stage, the OMS can frequently offer forms of assistance to the patient not available from other clinicians. Finally, the OMS can offer the patient the gift of relationship. This commitment may be the greatest gift and the greatest good that the OMS can offer the patient in the final stages of life.

PART II

End-of-life issues arise infrequently in the routine practice of oral and maxillofacial surgery. However, the OMS should understand the legal, ethical, and psychological issues that surround the treatment of patients who are facing death. Although these circumstances may arise abruptly because of trauma or an adverse anesthetic outcome, the focus of this discussion is the subset of the OMS's patients with progressive illness, leaving little or no hope of recovery. For the OMS who is involved in the management of patients with head and neck cancers, end-of-life issues are likely to be encountered quite often. In the United States, approximately 39,000 cases of cancer affecting the oral cavity, pharynx, and/or larynx are diagnosed each year.[10] Most are detected in the advanced stages, with regional spread and extensive local involvement. As such, the OMS is often faced with a tumor that is clinically compelling and may surmise the diagnosis and prognosis based on the history and physical examination even before the biopsy has taken place. Nonetheless, the role of the OMS in the continuous management of these patients is pivotal to providing comfort and care to the patient and family during the treatment and in the final stages of disease.

When the OMS is faced with a patient suffering from oral, esophageal, pharyngeal, or laryngeal cancer, medical decision-making may be facilitated by the use of a framework designed for this population. Thompson and Krouse[11] proposed 7 guiding principles that may be applied by the surgeon when discussing the treatment of a life-threatening condition with a patient and family members. These principles are as follows:

1. Be sure the patient and family understand the diagnosis and prognosis.
2. Set new treatment goals (for the patient as well as for the surgeon).
3. Assess new symptoms.
4. Discuss treatment options for the new symptom or symptoms.
5. Make a recommendation.
6. Never say "there is nothing to be done."
7. Do not abandon patients.

Open and honest communication may well be the most important element of care for the patient who may no longer benefit significantly from surgical, medical, or pharmacologic interventions. The OMS must ensure that patients and their families understand the significance of the disease as well as the potential risks and benefits of any proposed course of action. In a 1998 study involving focus groups consisting of patients, their families, and professionals providing care, patients reported receiving "too much information about the details of the surgical procedures but not enough information on the side effects of treatment or what to expect during and after treatment."[12] It is the duty of the OMS to discuss all options with the patient, including the nontreatment option and those that do not involve surgical treatment.

The surgeon should play an active role with the patient and the patient's family to set new treatment goals as the focus of care shifts from cure to palliation. As discussed previously, the wishes of the competent patient must always be honored. The principles of beneficence, nonmalfeasance, autonomy, veracity, fidelity, and proportionate versus disproportionate means must be upheld by the surgeon and the patient's family. A treatment plan is best developed and implemented when the clinician has a clear understanding of how much medical and surgical intervention is acceptable to the patient. Having an informed patient who provides definitive parameters also minimizes the stress and confusion for family members should their loved one become unable to make decisions independently. A detailed discussion of the patient's legal options is beyond the scope of this article; however, there are several terms with which the OMS should be familiar when preparing to discuss treatment options with the patient and family members.[13,14] Readers are encouraged to refer to the legislation set forth by their state regarding legal issues in medical care.

The advance directive is a legal document expressing the wishes of patients regarding issues that may arise when they are no longer able to make choices or communicate. The most common forms of advance directive are the power of attorney (POA/ health care proxy) and the living will. A POA is a document naming a person who will make all decisions regarding the patient's health care should the patient become unable to do so. A living will describes the patient's wishes and usually includes choices to be made given specific situations. *Comfort care only* refers to orders that include palliative measures but preclude active attempts to control the patient's disease. *Do not intubate* is an order that prohibits the use of endotracheal intubation and mechanical ventilation to support respiration. Because a tracheotomy bypasses normal pathways and requires ventilatory support, this option must be discussed in depth with the patient. *Do not resuscitate* indicates the patient choice to decline any measures to stop or reverse cardiac arrest, including defibrillation, intravenous fluids, blood products, and medications.

Beyond their role in ensuring that patients' end-of-life wishes are honored, advance directives provide a secondary benefit by reducing the financial burden on the already stretched health care system. In Claire H Altman's statement, A Proposal to Develop a National Strategy for End-of-Life Care That Reduces Cost and Increases Quality of Care, she provides statistics on spending patterns for terminally ill patients. She states: "Twenty-five percent of the annual Medicare budget of $627 billion is spent on care for persons in the last year of life, with 40% of that number spent in the last 30 days. Medical care at the end of life consumes 10–12% of the nation's total health care budget.[1] These numbers have not changed significantly over the last ten years despite the fact that in-patient, residential and home hospice care services are less costly and underutilized—and provide higher quality service. Existing data (mainly from the 1980's) suggest that hospice and advance directives can save between 25 and 40% of health care costs during the last month of life, with savings decreasing to 10–17% over the last six months of life.[2] The Congressional Budget Office forecasts that the cost of long term care will reach $207 billion in 2020 and $346 billion in 2040."[3,5]

Altman goes on to provide the reasons for end-of-life care having such a high cost. These include a general lack of knowledge regarding treatment options and support systems that are available and, frequently, the absence of advance directives designed to guide a family faced with these difficult choices. Proposed strategies for easing the burden on patients, families, and the health care system involve the education of health care providers on death and dying, including the ethical principles related to end-of-life care and the important role played by culture in medical decision-making. Cultural competency is a factor in all interactions between the clinician and those affected by medical treatment. At no other time in the life of a patient are cultural issues more critical than during the difficult hours, days, and months before death. These moments require extraordinary sensitivity and effective communication transcending ethnic, cultural, and language barriers. Additionally, financial incentives may be offered to hospitals providing advance directive education to patients and families. Medicare reimbursement for assisted-living programs for patients with terminal illness may decrease the frequency of hospitalizations and concurrent medical and surgical interventions that occur during the last years or months of the patient's life, thereby lowering costs. Although the process of early discussion and planning for end-of-life decisions does serve the greater good, the primary purpose is to afford each patient dignity, respect, and a voice at a time when those rights may be lost.

STRATEGIES FOR THE OMS

As the OMS continues to care for the terminally ill patient, each visit should include the assessment of any new symptoms and focus on treatment options for the relief of each symptom. Alleviation of pain and suffering should not be postponed to the last few weeks of the patient's life. Patients with cancer of the head and neck confront various unique physical and psychological challenges that may not be as predominant in patients with other types of cancers. Patients with head and neck cancer confront significant functional and quality-of-life issues, including chronic pain, changes in speech, alteration or loss of taste sensation, loss of teeth, difficulties with mastication and swallowing, and possible need for tube feeding and/or tracheostomy. The disease, its prognosis. and its treatment may also produce anxiety and depression.[15] Cancers of the oral cavity and associated structures often lead to facial disfigurement that profoundly affects the patient's self-image and, thus, self-esteem. Social interactions may become limited, compounding the isolation that patients may already feel. Specific palliative treatments available to the OMS have been described and may improve the quality of life for patients suffering from pain or discomfort secondary to oral and head and neck malignancies. Pain management is a critical issue in palliative care. Cancers affecting the head and neck region often infiltrate surrounding structures, such as cranial nerves, cervical plexus, sensory ganglia, and sympathetic trunks. The lingual nerve, mandibular branch of the trigeminal nerve, and glossopharyngeal nerve are most commonly responsible for chronic pain from head and neck cancer[16] The OMS should apply appropriate principles, ensure that selected analgesics are adequate, and consider consultation with a pain management specialist.

Head and neck tumors can grow to significant size thereby compromising the patient's airway. Debulking is a palliative surgical procedure that can be performed by the OMS in selected cases to reduce dysphagia and odynophagia.[13] The use of lasers may facilitate debulking of tumors that tend to be vascular, because the wound is coagulated while tissue is vaporized. The OMS may also be involved in the management of those carcinomas that have eroded facial soft tissues. Advanced lesions producing necrosis are terribly disfiguring and are often associated with a fetid odor, which decreases patients' willingness to socialize, worsening their feelings of isolation. Although wound care is a complex process, the OMS is still able to provide education to patients and their families regarding cleaning and dressing. If necessary, early consultation by a wound care specialist should also be sought.

Most oral and oropharyngeal cancers are detected after the tumor has become sizeable and regional lymphatics are involved. Thus, the combination of irradiation and surgery is often required, and the sequelae of irradiation typically compound the anatomic changes produced by the tumor and the surgical procedures used to address it and any associated lymph nodes. Xerostomia is a common and potentially devastating complication of radiotherapy. It profoundly affects the quality of life and is the underlying cause of many of the complications experienced by patients who have been treated for head and neck cancers. Radiation oncologists use various approaches intended to minimize damage to salivary glands. Surgical procedures with similar goals have also been described. Among these is the Seikaly-Jha procedure intended to preserve one submandibular gland by surgically transferring it to the submental space before radiation therapy.[13] Patients who have already undergone radiation therapy and report xerostomia are managed by increasing saliva production via mechanical, gustatory, or pharmacologic stimulation, by the use of saliva substitutes, and by adherence to a rigorous protocol of meticulous oral hygiene. Transcutaneous electric nerve stimulation has also produced encouraging results in increasing salivary flow from the parotid glands and in providing some pain relief.[13]

It is not uncommon for the terminally ill patient to feel overwhelmed by the volume and weight of the information being provided at the time of diagnosis and follow-up visits. The OMS should not hesitate to make recommendations based on the patient's goals of treatment. In fact, a study by Strauss[17] concluded that "most patients desired their surgeon to assume a closely supportive role" after surgery. By remaining active during the patient's disease trajectory, the OMS becomes a resource for palliative care that other medical specialists may not be able to provide. The OMS should make the patient feel that no matter how grave the prognosis, the surgeon will always do whatever is possible to minimize the negative impact of the disease and its treatment on the patient's quality of life. The OMS should provide assurance that while the disease may be incurable, something can always be done to make the patient more comfortable during this challenging time. The surgeon who continues to stay involved in the patient's care and remains a resource for the patient and family members is providing comfort. This may be more important than anything else and is associated with psychological benefit to the patient, the patient's family, and the clinician. It is not in the surgeon's nature to step back from definitive interventions and play a supportive role. Nonetheless, there is great satisfaction to be derived from having eased pain, provided comfort, and ensured dignity at the end of a patient's journey.

REFERENCES

1. Code of ethics and professionalism for orthopaedic surgeons. Rosemont (IL): American Academy Orthopaedic Surgeons; 2009.
2. Thomson AR, Krouse RS. Terminal care in head and neck cancer patients: a framework for medical decision making. J Am Coll Surg 2004;198(5):837–42.
3. Bridges J, Mulder J. End of life issues in terminal cancer. Oral Maxillofac Surg Clin North Am 2006; 18:643–5.
4. Assael LA. Managing chronic illnesses in the oral and maxillofacial surgery practice. J Oral Maxillofac Surg 2009;67:243–4.
5. Brody H. The physician-patient relationship. In: Veatch R, editor. Medical ethics. 2nd edition. Sudbury (MA): Jones and Bartlett Publishers; 1997. p. 75–101.
6. Daugherty CK, Hlubocky FJ. What are terminally ill cancer patients told about their expected deaths? A study of cancer physicians' self-reports of prognosis disclosure. J Clin Oncol 2008;26(36): 5988–93.
7. Oken D. What to tell cancer patients: a study of physician attitudes. JAMA 1961;175:1120–8.
8. Code of medical ethics of the American Medical Association, Council on judicial and ethical affairs, 2008–2009. Chicago. Ethics manual, ethics and human rights committee. 5th edition. Philadelphia, Pennsylania: American College of Physicians; 2009.
9. Annas GJ. Standard of are: the law of American bioethics. New York: Oxford University Press; 1993.
10. Bridges Mulder J. End of life issues in oral cancer. Oral Maxillofac Surg Clin North Am 2006;18:643–5.

11. Thompson AR, Krouse RS. Terminal care in head and neck cancer patients: a framework for medical decision making. J Am Coll Surg 2004;198(5): 837–41.

12. Edwards D. Head and neck cancer services: views of patients, their families and professionals. Br J Oral Maxillofac Surg 1998;36:99–102.

13. Elackattu A, Jalisi S. Living with head and neck cancer and coping with dying when treatments fail. Otolaryngol Clin North Am 2009;42:171–84.

14. Altman, Claire. Proposal to develop a national strategy for end-of-life care that reduces cost and increases quality of care. Statement of testimony before U.S. house of representatives ways and means committee. April 16, 2009.

15. Penner J. Psychosocial care of patients with head and neck cancer. Semin Oncol Nurs 2009;25(3): 231–41.

16. Fortunato L, Ridge JA. Surgical palliation of head and neck cancer. Curr Probl Cancer 1995;19(3): 153–65.

17. Strauss R. Psychosocial responses to oral and maxillofacial surgery for head and neck cancer. J Oral Maxillofac Surg 1989;47:343–8.

Substance Abuse Issues in Oral and Maxillofacial Practice

Robert J. DeFalco, DDS[a,b,]*, Michael Erlichman, DDS[a,b],
Sharang Tickoo[c], Steven D. Passik, PhD[c,d]

KEYWORDS
- Substance abuse • Addiction
- Oral and maxillofacial surgery • Drug abuse

Addiction is extremely common in the United States. Because addiction has a lifetime prevalence in adults of 15% in this country, oral and maxillofacial surgeons will inevitably encounter patients with addictions. Treatment of these patients is complicated in many ways by their problems with adherence, poor overall health and dental status, and, most importantly, management of pain. Further complicating the issue of proper pain management is the growing problem of prescription drug abuse. The focus of most drug abuse these days has become prescription opioids. Oral and maxillofacial surgeons are likely to encounter people with addictions who are abusing commonly used opioids in oral and maxillofacial practice, or those seeking these drugs for diversion (illegal resale). Oral and maxillofacial surgeons are often called on to manage acute pain in patients with whom they do not have a longstanding relationship; as a result, their history of abuse may not be known to the clinician. Additionally, oral and maxillofacial surgeons frequently manage chronic pain in which opioid therapy may be a component. Thus, these surgeons must learn how to identify addictions and manage their complications in oral and maxillofacial surgical situations.

Additional prevalence data further drive home the ubiquity of this problem. Worldwide, an 16 million people use injectable drugs.[1] Almost one-third of adults in the United States meet the criteria for an alcohol use disorder at some point in their lives.[2] In 2000, excessive alcohol use led to 85,000 premature deaths within the United States.[3] In 2003, 34.9 million people in the United States had admitted to using cocaine.[4] The cost of addictive illness in the United States is estimated to be $144 billion annually in health care and job loss. Substance abuse is greatest in individuals between ages 18 and 25 years. It is more common in men than in women, and greater in residents in urban areas than in rural locations. Addicted individuals comprise an average of 20% of patients in general medical facilities and 35% in general psychiatric units.[5]

Substance-related disorders are conditions in which an individual uses or abuses a substance that leads to maladaptive behaviors or symptoms. These disorders can be separated into substance dependence and substance abuse.[1] Substance abuse refers to a maladaptive pattern of substance use leading to clinically significant impairment or distress, manifested by at least one symptom that interferes with life functioning within a 12-month period. Substance dependence requires at least three of the following within a 12-month period: development of tolerance to the substance, withdrawal symptoms, persistent

[a] St Joseph's Regional Medical Center, Department of Oral and Maxillofacial Surgery, 703 Main Street, Paterson, NJ 07503, USA
[b] Seton Hall University School of Health and Medical Sciences, 400 South Orange Avenue, South Orange, NJ 07079, USA
[c] Department of Psychiatry and Behavioral Sciences, Memorial Sloan Kettering Cancer Center, 160 East 53rd Street, New York, NY 10022, USA
[d] Department of Psychiatry, Weill-Cornell Medical Center, 1300 York Avenue, New York, NY 10065, USA
* Corresponding author. 30 West Century Road, Suite 210, Paramus, NJ 07562.
E-mail address: bobdefl@aol.com

Oral Maxillofacial Surg Clin N Am 22 (2010) 527–535
doi:10.1016/j.coms.2010.07.011

desire and unsuccessful attempts to stop the substance, ingestion of larger amounts of the substance than intended, diminished life functioning, and persistent substance use in the phase of physical or psychological problems.

More than 50% (and in at least one study, more than 85%) of people with substance-related disorders have comorbid non–substance-related psychiatric disorders. They are usually termed *dual diagnosis* individuals. Comorbid psychiatric diagnoses include depression, personality disorders, anxiety disorder, and dysthymia.[5]

ADDICTION MEDICINE 101 FOR ORAL AND MAXILLOFACIAL SURGEONS

The American Society of Addiction Medicine (ASAM), American Pain Society (APS), and American Academy of Pain Medicine (AAPM) define addiction as a primary, chronic, neurobiological disease with genetic, psychosocial, and environmental factors influencing its development and manifestations.[6] In people with these predisposing factors (genetic, psychosocial, environmental), single exposures to addictive substances may produce permanent changes in the brain, affecting memory, and can create a process of pathologic learning, specifically a craving for drugs. Once drug use becomes excessive, disturbances in the stress response system lead to compulsive repetitive patterns in an effort to capture the initial reinforcement or block withdrawal. The end result is repetitive behaviors in the face of negative consequences, which are complicated by denial. Denial is a complex defense mechanism that typically accompanies addictive disease. These individuals are often convinced they do not have the disease, sometimes even in the face of overwhelming evidence to the contrary.[7] Clinicians can remember the symptoms of addiction using the mnemonic device of the 4 C's: Compulsive use, continuing use in the face of negative repercussions, loss of control, and cravings (**Table 1**).

Genetics

Familial transmission has been proven in alcoholism. Family illness, twin, and adoptive studies have all supported a genetic predisposition. What has been shown in alcoholism has generally held true for other substances and addictive behaviors.[8,9] Strong evidence shows that the development of addiction to drugs of abuse is partly a function of predisposing factors in an individual's genome and factors associated with childhood and adolescent development.[10] Thus, although a widely held viewpoint is that drug addiction is a form of moral weakness, it is vital

Table 1
Behavioral criteria indicative of addiction (the 4 C's)

Criteria	Specific Suggestive Observable Behaviors
Control over use impaired	Frequent claims of "lost" or "stolen" medicines, signs of withdrawal
Compulsion to use	A feeling of inability to stop use, multiple failed attempts to stop use
Continuing use despite harm from use	Frequent intoxication, impairment of function, damage to physical, social, and mental status
Craving of the substance	Strong urge to acquire and use the substance, particularly after peak subsides

that this misconception be dispelled so that addiction may be treated as what it truly is: as a disease for which vulnerability may be inherited.

Reward

The reward system of the brain involves the mesolimbic dopamine system. These pathways control the automatic bodily functions of the brain stem and peripheral nervous system, and the emotional or limbic areas of the brain to the prefrontal cortex, which is the thinking or reflective and decision-making part of the central nervous system. Neurotransmitters such as dopamine and ß-endorphins facilitate the communication of these different systems in the reward center. This pathway, which is altered in the addict, is involved in essential behaviors, such as eating, sleeping, and sex. The addict's initial motivation is to feel pleasure; as the substances of abuse stimulate this reward pathway, the addict's focus shifts from these essential behaviors toward their substances. In the pursuit of reward, the receptors that naturally mediate reward become desensitized, creating the need for more substance contributing to tolerance and withdrawal, which ultimately leads to addiction.[11]

Learning and memory are modified by addictive behaviors; they usually shape survival behaviors related to rewards. As their cognitive processes treat the acquisition of a substance of abuse as a reward, this substance becomes as appealing as other essential activities. This process results in the shift from drug use to drug abuse in the form of a compulsion as strong as other basic drives, such as hunger. Addicts are forced by their minds to think of a drug as equally important as food; their craving becomes analogous to the sensations associated with starvation and thirst.[10]

Motivation

Motivation is a key component in recovery. Early in treatment, the patient may experience a lack of concentration, irritability, and insomnia, referred to as post−acute withdrawal. During this phase, the patient has a tendency to return to the addictive habit, and affected individuals will require physiologic, psychological, and social support.

Given the reprogrammed circuitry in the brains of those suffering from addiction, initiating and maintaining motivation may be difficult. Kalivas and Volkow[12] proposed that with addiction, a deregulation occurs in the motivation center of the brain, which is reorganized to establish behaviors that support substance-seeking and abuse. This reorganization produces a cycle of behavior that becomes increasingly difficult to break.

Clinical Presentation

Although some of the signs and symptoms of abuse and addiction are universal, specific manifestations are associated with each of the commonly abused substances. The substances with most relevance to oral and maxillofacial surgery (OMS) are reviewed here.

Alcohol is relevant to the oral and maxillofacial surgeon simply by virtue of its prevalence. In addition, alcoholics are prone to excessive bleeding during surgeries. Alcohol is the most commonly abused substance in the United States, with up to 15% of the population having abused or been dependent on alcohol at some time in their lives. Behavioral changes include expansive mood, social withdrawal, mood liability, irritability, and aggression. Physical and neurologic symptoms include decreased concentration, attention, and coordination. Alcohol abusers also tend to be impulsive and exhibit impaired judgement.[5] Withdrawals begin 4 to 12 hours after the last consumed drink and are associated with symptoms such as tremor, tachycardia, increased blood pressure, anxiety, and diaphoresis. Withdrawals may last up to 5 days and be accompanied by seizures. Delirium tremens (DTs) occur in approximately 5% of these cases, and may be fatal. Chronic long-term users may develop Wernicke encephalopathy and Korsakoff syndrome. Wernicke encephalopathy is related to a thiamine deficiency and may be reversible with replacement. Korsakoff psychosis affects the areas of the brain involved with memory.

Sedative hypnotics affect the central nervous system. These prescription drugs are used in many different clinical situations, including those encountered by oral and maxillofacial surgeons, and include the benzodiazepines, barbiturates, chloral hydrate, and meprobamate. An improved ability to initiate and maintain sleep and a decrease in agitation and anxiety are desirable effects of most of these agents, but these effects may also lead to misuse. Misuse can also produce hypotension, impairments in balance, speech changes, central nervous system depression, and respiratory depression. Drug tolerance is also commonplace and leads to increasing demand for the drug, and ultimately the potential for addiction. Unlike abused substances procured illegally, these medications are generally prescribed by physicians and dentists. As with all potentially dangerous and controlled substances, the use of sedative-hypnotics should be carefully monitored by prescribers. Withdrawal reactions include anxiety, restlessness, gastrointestinal disturbance, hypotension, tachycardia, tremor, agitation, and, in severe cases, possibly seizures.[5]

Tobacco is smoked in cigarettes, pipes, and cigars and is also applied to the oral mucosa. Tobacco is a significant factor in the development of numerous diseases. Smoking tobacco is responsible for 20% of all deaths in the United States, including cardiovascular disease and many cancers. Although other elements of tobacco smoke are carcinogenic and generally damaging, nicotine is the active ingredient associated with dependence. The average age at which smokers begin is 15 years, and approximately one-quarter of the adult United States population engages in this habit. For long-term users who attempt smoking cessation, withdrawals usually occur within 24 hours and are characterized by depression , insomnia, irritability, anxiety, restlessness, decreased concentration, decreased heart rate, increased appetite, and increased weight.

Particularly relevant to the oral and maxillofacial surgeon is the opioid and opiate class of drugs. The term *opiates* refers to substances derived from opium alkaloids, whereas *opioids* are substances synthesized to have similar effects. Widely prescribed for pain management, opiates and opioids are often packaged as combination agents with peripheral analgesics. The principal effects of these drugs are euphoria, analgesia, and sedation. Other effects include respiratory depression, pupillary constriction, nausea and vomiting, constipation, pruritis, and dysphoria.

Tolerance and addiction may occur quickly with this class of drugs, presenting great difficulties given the frequent need for short-acting opioids in patients recovering from surgeries. Withdrawal begins rapidly after the last use, and is characterized by anxiety, sweating, tremor, agitation, gastrointestinal disturbance, and dehydration. Withdrawal may be a protracted process lasting up to 2 weeks.

Although heroin is the most commonly used illicit drug in this class and was responsible for 45% of all drug-related deaths in 1993, prescription opioids are the most relevant to the oral and maxillofacial surgeon. The fact that pain in surgery patients must be appropriately managed necessitates the prescription of these opioids. However, the addictive potential of opioids must also be elucidated and managed.

In a 2006 study, 51 of 109 (47%) persons presenting for treatment of oxycodone addiction were first exposed to opioids through a prescription for pain.[13] From 2002 to 2005, a total of 9.4 billion doses of opioids were prescribed,[14] and it is no coincidence that at the end of 2005, opioids displaced marijuana as the new illicit drug of choice for the first time.[15] Even when a patient is not the one abusing the opioid, another member of the household may be misappropriating the drug for misuse or even sale. For example, an older patient who is continually complaining of pain and asking for renewals may be the unwitting victim of a visiting grandchild who is diverting the medication. Nearly 70% of people who use opioids recreationally receive them from friends and family. College-aged women are the fastest-growing subgroup of nonmedical users of opioids in the country. At the very least, cautious use of opioids requires education regarding proper drug storage and the dangers of sharing these medications. In this article's section on pain management, a range of strategic suggestions will be offered for how to safely plan opioid therapy. When prescribing opioid medications for postoperative pain, quantity must be an important consideration. It is not desirable to mask the symptoms of a true complication by the prolonged use of opioid analgesics. Moreover, unused medications that remain in the household long after the patient's need is gone are a significant potential hazard.

SUBSTANCE ABUSE TREATMENT

Individuals who abuse substances often have underlying or associated psychological disorders that must also be diagnosed properly and treated along with the addiction. Treatment is generally divided into three realms: acute intoxication/overdose, withdrawal, and rehabilitation. Pharmacologic and psychological treatment modalities are available, and when these are combined appropriately, patients may be more successful at maintaining abstinence.[5]

Alcohol intoxication may be severe and is associated with respiratory depression, coma, or death. Initial supportive therapy may be required. Withdrawal will begin from a couple of hours to days from the last drink. Approximately 5% of the people will develop DT's, which will lead to death in 1% to 5% of the cases. Benzodiazepines are commonly used to treat the symptoms of withdrawal and as prophylaxis against DTs. In more severe cases, phenobarbital may be used. During acute withdrawal, alcoholics will often require rehydration, with normal saline being the preferred fluid. The patient's electrolytes should be closely monitored and thiamine should be administered along with folate to help reverse Wernicke encephalopathy. Thiamine is much less likely to improve the cognitive impairment and memory loss associated with Korsakoff. In a certain population of patients, the use of antipsychotics may be necessary.[16]

It is widely believed that the most successful way to end alcohol abuse and dependence is for the user to commit to complete abstinence. Individuals who commit to abstinence may benefit from medications that may assist in their recovery. Naltrexone, disulfiram, acamprosate, and topiramate have all been shown to help motivated patients with their recovery. Using these agents in conjunction with nonpharmacologic therapy through an addiction specialist or an established program has been shown to be effective in patient recovery.[17]

Patients experiencing opiate/opioid intoxication usually present with severe respiratory distress and may have pressure nerve palsies from extended periods of immobility, and hypotension and aspiration-related problems.[18] Initial management of these patients focuses on airway control to avoid hypoxia and aspiration. Naloxone, 0.4 to 2 mg, is the preferred drug as a reversal, but it is important to monitor the patient because the half-life of the naloxone may be shorter than the substance used and the patient may experience relapse. Withdrawal from opiates or opioids usually occurs within hours of the last dose and initial treatment focuses on management of the acute withdrawal symptoms. These symptoms are usually controlled with decreasing doses of long-acting opioid antagonists, such as methadone or buprenorphine. The use of clonidine three times a day may also be helpful, and agitation may be controlled with benzodiazepines.

Many patients do not tolerate detoxification well and relapse quickly. Maintenance programs may be a better alternative because the patient is less likely to relapse.[3] Psychotherapeutic management also may be of value. Pain management in this population of patients seems to be an issue, especially after surgical procedures. For patients in methadone maintenance programs, the general recommendation is that the usual methadone regimen be continued and supplemented by nonsteroidal anti-inflammatory drugs, if possible. For severe pain, narcotic analgesics may be required, but the patient is likely to require higher dosages, and programmatic restrictions relative to the use of prescribed medications may exist.[19,20]

Treatment of sedative hypnotic overdoses depends on the drug used and route of administration. Furthermore, treatment is complicated considerably by the concurrent self-administration of other substances, as happens often. Respiratory and cardiac consequences are common, and management follows standard protocols. The severity of withdrawal depends on the dosage and duration of use. Strategies for withdrawal usually center on gradual dosage reduction or substitution with a long-term benzodiazepine or phenobarbital, and then proceed to tapering dosage. The rate of taper should be tailored to each patient, and again, psychotherapy should be used; these interventions tend to be extremely effective in long-term treatment.

Benzodiazepines cause central nervous system depression, hypotension, and respiratory depression. Supportive measures must be used and, when indicated, flumazenil should be used to reverse the benzodiazepine. As the clinical duration of action of many benzodiazepines exceeds that of flumazenil, multiple doses may be required with an extended period of careful patient monitoring. Withdrawal symptoms include anxiety, tremor, insomnia, fever, tinnitus, nausea, myalgias, vomiting, seizures, and diaphoresis. In the case of severe withdrawals, it may be necessary to reinstitute a benzodiazepine and taper the dose down slowly.

Treatment of stimulant overdosage involves management of the central nervous system symptoms and autonomic hyperactivity. Cooling, hydration, and monitoring are paramount. Withdrawals are managed symptomatically, although antipsychotics and antidepressants may be useful. Psychotherapy is a vital component of any approach likely to achieve good long-term outcomes.

Nicotine intoxication is extremely rare, but when it does occur, it is usually associated with replacement therapy used by those in the process of smoking cessation. Withdrawals begin within 6 hours of cessation and symptoms may last up to 6 weeks. Findings include slowing of the EEG, cravings, a decreased metabolic rate, and a decrease in heart rate. The increased levels of nicotine may displace the protein-binding of other medications, thereby making more of the drug readily available. Most successful treatment therapies include both psychosocial counseling and pharmacologic intervention. Even with all of these therapies, absolute cessation rate remains at only 20%.[21]

THE INTERFACE OF OMS PAIN MANAGEMENT AND ADDICTION

Obviously, the solution to the problem of pain in the OMS setting is not the total avoidance of opioid medications. As essential tools in the fight against pain, such effective medicines enhance the lives of many patients and are the cornerstone of the treatment of acute postoperative pain and play a prominent role in the management of chronic pain. However, because of the inherent risks in the abuse of this class of drugs (with estimates as high as 1 in 5 doses being diverted for black-market resale), certain precautions must be taken. Oral and maxillofacial surgeons face various issues that confound pain management that other medical professionals do not Oral and maxillofacial surgeons often treat acute and postoperative pain, requiring them to prescribe opioids to patients whose drug abuse histories are not known because a long-standing doctor–patient relationship usually does not exist.

Screening

To assist oral and maxillofacial surgeons in prescribing opioids, several screening tools help to identify high-risk patients. These tools have been preliminarily validated in pain clinic settings, and although no empirical data exist on their use in OMS settings, they may have use.

The first of these tools is the Screener and Opioid Assessment for Patients with Pain (SOAPP). Containing only 14 items and using a 5-point scale (from 0 meaning "never" to 4 meaning "very often"), this screening tool can be completed by patients while they are in the waiting room. Although the available data are correlational and not causal in nature, SOAPP is actively being researched and has high potential to emerge as a clinically relevant tool. The scores from each item are summed, and a relatively low cutoff score (8) exists to account for the underreporting of behaviors.

The Opioid Risk Tool (ORT) is a questionnaire consisting of five yes-or-no questions. It covers social issues that may indicate a predisposition to addiction, such as family and personal history of substance abuse or psychological disease. Patients can complete it in the waiting room or a clinician form can be completed during the patient visit as part of the patient intake. Each positive response is associated with a different score based on patient gender (ie, a family history of alcoholism is worth 3 points for male patients and 1 for female) and the point totals are summed up. "Low risk" is defined as scores of 3 or less, whereas scores of 8 or more indicate a high risk of addiction. When tested on 185 consecutive patients, it showed very good ability to predict which patients would go on to abuse or become addicted to medications with c statistic values of 0.82 for men and 0.85 for women. A risk of the ORT is the brief face-value nature of its questions; any deception on the patient's part severely compromises the ORT's ability to screen for moderate- or high-risk patients.[22]

Ongoing Monitoring in Patients With Chronic Pain on Opioids

Four major domains exist in which the efficacy of opioid therapy in the treatment of chronic pain may be considered. These four A's—analgesia, activities of daily living, aberrant drug related behaviors, and adverse effects—determine whether opioid therapy remains a good choice for a patient. Of the four, aberrant drug-related behaviors are the signs that should be most carefully monitored to determine whether a patient with chronic pain may be losing control and in danger of addiction to their opioids. These behaviors can include mild signs that may not be cause for alarm, such as unkempt appearance or occasional dose escalation. However, more extreme behavior, such as changing the route of administration or constant requests for early renewals, most certainly must be addressed. Every follow-up note written on the OMS patient on chronic opioid therapy should contain a mention of all four domains of outcome.

When Noncompliance Occurs: The Differential Diagnosis of Aberrant Drug Related Behaviors

Aberrant behaviors are common in people with pain who are taking opioids. Determining the meaning of these behaviors involves trying to understand the motive behind them. These behaviors may be a sign of pseudo-addiction, not addiction. When a patient aggressively requests higher doses or escalates the dose unilaterally, this may be a sign of untreated or undertreated pain. In pseudo-addiction, behavior is driven by inadequate analgesia, and these behaviors resolve when the patient is treated properly. Addiction,

on the other hand, is characterized by uncontrollable behaviors that do not resolve, even with increased doses. Distinguishing between the two makes for a very perplexing differential diagnosis, whereas misdiagnosing these behaviors can have extreme negative ramifications and result in the suffering of a patient. However, problematic behaviors from pseudo-addiction rarely imply criminal intent, such as when patients report pain but intend to sell or divert medications. Generally, patients will describe uncontrolled pain rather than loss of control from their perspective. Thus, clinicians often have to "walk the line" between the two possibilities by beginning the process of imposing limits while titrating drugs upward to effect until the behavior comes under control or escalates further before the diagnosis is clinched.

Other potential causes of noncompliant behavior also exist. Untreated psychiatric comorbidities can drive aberrant drug-related behavior. For example, patients with extreme anxiety about OMS procedures may overuse their pain medications for the treatment of anxiety or panic. Referral to mental health professionals may be an important way to obviate the need to overuse pain medications for the self-medication of psychological problems.

Finally, drug diversion may explain behaviors such as repeated requests for early renewals. Urine toxicology screening showing absence of the metabolites of pain medications that the oral and maxillofacial surgeon is prescribing may help identify this as a clinical issue.

Management of Risk: The Risk Management Package in Chronic Opioid Therapy

Passik[23] has elsewhere described the so-called risk management package in chronic opioid therapy (**Box 1**). It is important for the oral and

---

Box 1
Risk management package that should be considered for patients undergoing opioid therapy

Screening and risk stratification

Use of Prescription Monitoring Program data

Compliance monitoring

   Urine drug testing

   Pill/patch counts

Education about drug storage and sharing

Psychotherapy and highly structured approaches

Abuse-deterrent/-resistant strategies in opioid formulation

maxillofacial surgeon to recognize that the paradigm in chronic pain management with opioids has been changing, partially in response to the problems encountered regarding prescription drug abuse. A range of clinical strategies for delivering opioid therapy in a tailored fashion for patients at various degrees of risk for opioid abuse is beyond the scope of this article, but are summarized in **Box 1**. The process begins with screening and risk stratification and proceeds to include a range of monitoring tools, including periodic urine drug screening and consultation with mental health and addiction professionals.

Special Note on the Methadone-Maintained Patient and the Patient in Recovery

Within the addiction community a folklore exists, much of which probably describes actual clinical practice, in which misconceptions about methadone-maintained patients and their need for pain management in the OMS setting has led to immense suffering in this patient population. Perhaps the most common misconception is that the methadone-maintained patient requires no analgesics for acute pain. If anything, some recent work has described a decreased pain threshold for people maintained for methadone.[24] Thus, patients who undergo OMS procedures will require opioids as any other patient would, and perhaps in higher doses because of either their tolerance or this decreased pain threshold. Consultation with professionals in pain management or methadone maintenance may be helpful.

Addicts in recovery who present for OMS procedures are likely to express a reticence about exposure to opioids for their acute pain. Although in some instances nonopioid alternatives may be viable, these patients will require reassurance and help in maintaining control over their medicines if opioids are used. Some of their fears can be allayed in this fashion, although it is often important to remind these patients that untreated pain could be a stimulus for illicit drug use and relapse in and of itself. Again, consultation with professionals in pain management or addiction may be helpful in planning these patients' postoperative pain management.

PROFESSIONAL AND ETHICAL CONSIDERATIONS IN THE DETECTION OF IMPAIRED COLLEAGUES

The American Medical Association (AMA) defines an impaired physician as one who is unable to fulfill professional or personal responsibilities because of psychiatric illness, alcoholism, or drug dependency, An estimated 10% to 15% of physicians become impaired at some point during their careers.[25–28] These rates of substance abuse and dependence are comparable to the general population. Addiction is a disease with genetic, psychiatric, and social components, often aggravated by stress. Academic success, intellect, and the achievement of professional credentials do not preclude the possibility of addiction. Given the stresses of a medical career, the access to controlled substances, and the genetic basis of the disease, medical professionals are unsurprisingly among the most vulnerable to this disease.

Identification of the impaired health care professional is essential because patient well-being may be at stake, and untreated impairment may result in loss of license, health problems, and even death. Because health care professionals protect their workplace performance and image, identification of impaired individuals in this population and imposing intervention are difficult.[29,30] Detecting an impaired colleague is challenging and difficult because the signs and symptoms may be subtle and well-concealed.[31] Changes in personality, behavior, and physical appearance may be observed in the workplace. Personality changes may manifest in statements indicating distress, and signs of sadness, anxiety, or irritability may be noted. Outbreaks of anger or hostility toward colleagues, employees, or family also may be seen. Absenteeism and a decline in work performance and quality and may be noted along with an increase in patient and staff complaints at the office or hospital. In addition, signs may be present of heavy drinking, irritability, anger outbursts, sexual promiscuity, and possible citations for driving under the influence. Red flags include prescription writing for narcotics, stimulants, or sedatives for self or the office staff, and requesting prescriptions from colleagues for narcotics, stimulants, or sedatives. Abusers may look for ways to divert their patients' narcotics, stimulants, or sedatives for self use. Patient records may show an unusual pattern of prescribing drugs or inappropriate orders.

A deterioration of appearance, visible changes in weight, excessive fatigue, sleepiness, or obvious signs such as ataxic gait, slurred speech, unexplained tremor, needle marks, bandages, or alcohol on the breath may be noted. The doctor may request to personally administer drugs to patients. When on call, the impaired physician may be consistently unreachable or might be seen rounding on patients at odd hours.[32]

A history of progression may be noted, with use beginning in college and continuing through medical/dental school and residency. Initially, substance abuse may begin recreationally in professional school, where performance enhancement and self-medicating for pain, anxiety, or stress may also be seen. Over time, family and community life are impacted and financial issues may arise along with spiritual and emotional problems. Ultimately, physical health may decline, with job performance often affected last. Social, family, and emotional problems typically occur before the impairment of one's professional ability. Coombs[33] stated that professionals have an "artificial immunity" to addiction because of their high social standing and the misconception that professionals will somehow overcome these problems before they become too serious.[34]

Therefore, a major issue of concern with impaired health care professionals is the delay in detection. These abusers often engage in malignant denial, exhibiting the "I can take care of myself" attitude. Robert Coombs placed the drug-impaired into a category of "pedestal professionals," which include physicians, dentists, nurses, pharmacists, attorneys, and airline pilots for whom drug impairment is a problem, because each of these groups, as he says, is "trusted with our well being".[34]

Health care professionals have a duty and an obligation to report any good faith suspicion or concern about an impaired colleague. Reporting is not only an ethical obligation but also mandated by federal and state law and often by professional association codes and hospital bylaws. The AMA, American Dental Association, and American Association of Oral and Maxillofacial Surgeons (AAOMS) all have codes concerning the impaired health care professional. The AAOMS Code of Professional Conduct states that it is unethical for an oral and maxillofacial surgeon to practice while abusing controlled substances, alcohol, or other chemical agents that impair their ability to practice. The Code also requires all AAOMS members to urge impaired colleagues to seek treatment, and to report impairment to the well-being or equivalent committee of the state dental or medical board if they have first-hand knowledge of the colleague practicing while impaired.[35] A conspiracy of silence may delay intervention, with denial being the major obstacle to timely reporting and intervention. Fear that one's reputation may be damaged from reporting the impairment of a colleague, associate, or friend may be more powerful than the motivation to help the impaired individual and his or her patients.

The fear and intimidation that may prevent a clinician from exposing an impaired colleague stem from the possibility of destroying a career or the threat of legal retaliation. A reader's survey published in *Medical Economics* in an article entitled "Impaired Physicians: Speak no evil?" asked three questions: "1. What would you do if you became aware that a physician colleague was impaired by drugs, alcohol, or a physical or metal illness that could effect job performance or judgment?; 2. Is there an ethical obligation for you to take some action against an impaired colleague?; 3. Have you ever referred a patient to a physician in your group or managed care network even though you had concerns about that physician's suitability?" Two-thirds of physicians stated that they would report the doctor to the appropriate authorities in response to the first question.[36] The remainder stated that they would speak with the doctor privately but take no further action. The second question produced an almost unanimous response with little disagreement about the existence of an ethical obligation. As for referring to a potentially "unsuitable" colleague, 80% of respondents stated that they would not do so. Paul Root Wolpe, a bioethicist, evaluated the findings and commented on their accuracy.[36] He believed that physicians were not likely to report their colleagues to the authorities unless the person caused a problem with a patient.[36] It is important to use good judgment when considering a pattern of behavior rather than any isolated signs.[34] Clinicians share an ethical obligation to assist impaired colleagues and guide them to appropriate counseling and treatment. Clinicians are ethically bound to make every effort to prevent harm to the patients, family, friends, and associates of an impaired colleague. Perhaps a clinician's greatest obligation is to the individual.

SUMMARY

Substance abuse has far-reaching consequences for individuals, their families, and the community. Medications with abuse potential play an important role in the management of pain and are widely prescribed by the oral and maxillofacial surgeon. Reducing the likelihood of abuse and providing appropriate pain management for the known abuser are critical aspects of perioperative patient management. Health care providers are not immune to substance abuse and may, in fact, be at an elevated risk. Identification of impaired providers is essential to help them find the appropriate treatment and counseling and to prevent harm to their patients, family, friends, or associates.

REFERENCES

1. Leikin J. Substance related disorders in adults, DM. Dis Mon 2007;53(6):313–35.

2. Dawson DA, Li TK, Grant BF. A prospective study of risk drinking: at risk for what? Drug Alcohol Depend. 2008;95(1–2):62–72.

3. Mokakd AH, Marks JS, Stroup DF, et al. Actual cases of death In the United States, 2000. JAMA 2004;291(10):1238–45.

4. Afonso L, Mohammad T, Thatai D. Crack whips the heart: a review of the cardiovascular toxicity of cocaine. Am J of Cardiol 2007;100:1040–3.

5. Haber PS, Demirkol A, Lange K, et al. Management of injection drug users admitted to the hospital. Lancet 2009;374:1284–93.

6. Available at: http://www.ampainsoc.org/advocacy/opioids2.htm. Accessed July 29, 2010.

7. Koob G, Kreek J. Stress dysregulation of drug reward pathway, and the transition to drug dependence. Am J Psyhchiatry 2007;164:1149–61.

8. Van den Wildenberg E, Wiers RW, Dessers J, et al. A functional polymorphism of the mu receptor gene influences cue induced craving for alcohol in male heavy drinkers. Alcohol Clin Exp Res 2007; 31:1–10.

9. National Institute on Alcohol Abuse and Alcoholism. Alcohol alert. Genetics Of Alcoholism. Available at: http://pubs.niaaa.nih.gov/publications/aa60.htm. Accessed August 19, 2010.

10. Kalivas P. Predisposition to addiction: pharmacokinetics, pharmacodynamics, and brain circuitry. Am J Psychiatry 2003;160:1.

11. Angres DH, Angres KB. The disease of addiction: origins, treatment, and recovery. Dis Mon 2008;54: 696–721.

12. Kalivas PW, Volkow ND. The neural basis of addiction: a pathology of motivation and choice. Am J Psychiatry 2005;162:1403–13.

13. Passik SD, Hays L, Eisner N, et al. Psychiatric and pain characteristics of prescription drug abusers entering drug rehabilitation. J Pain Palliative Care Pharmacother 2006;20(2):5–13.

14. United States Department of Health and Human Services. The national survey on drug use and health (NSDUH) report: patterns and trends in nonmedical prescription pain reliever use: 2002 to 2005. Available at: http://www.oas.samhsa.gov/2k7/pain/pain.htm. Accessed July 29, 2010.

15. SAMHSA. Office of Applied Studies. 2005 National Survey on Drug Use and Health: National Findings. Available at: http://www.oas.samhsa.gov/NSDUH/2k5NSDUH/2k5results.htm#TOC. Accessed August 19, 2010.

16. Olmedo R, Hoffman RS. Withdrawal syndromes. Emerg Med North Amer 2000;18(2):273–88.

17. Willenbring M, Massey S, Gardner M. Helping patients who drink too much: an evidenced-based guide for primary care physicians. Am Fam Physician 2009;80(1):44–50.

18. Crowe AV, Howse M, Bell GM, et al. Substance abuse and the kidney. QJM 2000;93:147–52.

19. Mehta V, Langford RM. Acute pain management for opioid dependent patients. Anaesthesia 2006;61: 269–76.

20. Alford DP, Compton P, Samet JH. Acute pain management for patients receiving maintenance methadone or buprenorphine therapy. Ann Intern Med 2006;144:127–34.

21. Hatsukami D, Stead L, Gupta P. Tobacco addiction. J Lancet 2008;371:2027–38.

22. Passik SD, Kirsh KL. The interface between pain and drug abuse and the evolution of strategies to optimize pain management while minimizing drug abuse. Exp Clin Psychopharmacol 2008;16(5): 400–4.

23. Passik D. Issues in long-term opioid therapy: unmet needs, risks, and solutions. Mayo Clin Proc 2009; 84(7):593–601.

24. Compton MA. Cold-pressor pain tolerance in opiate and cocaine abusers: correlates of drug abuse type and use status. J Pain Symptom Manage 1994;9: 462–73.

25. Markel H. The accidental addict (editorial). N Engl J Med 2005;352(10):966–8.

26. Brewster JM. Prevalence of alcohol and other drug problems among physicians. JAMA 1986;255(14): 1913–20.

27. Berge KH, Seppala MD, Schipper AM. Chemical dependency and the physician. Mayo Clin Proc 2009;84(7):625–31.

28. Hughes PH, Brandenburg N, et al. Prevalence of substance abuse among US physicians. JAMA 1992;267(17):2333–9.

29. Baldisseri MR. Impaired healthcare professional. Crit Care Med 2007;35(Suppl 2):S106–16.

30. Cicala RS. Substance abuse among physicians: what you need to know. Hosp Physician 2003; 39(7):39–46.

31. Monahan G. Drug use/misuse among health professionals. Subst Use Misuse 2003;38(11–13): 1877–81.

32. Boisaubin EV, Levine RE. Identifying and assisting the impaired physician. Am J Med Sci 2001;322(1): 31–6.

33. Coombs RH. Drug-Impaired Professionals. Cambridge, Mass: Harvard University Press; 1997. p. 351. ISBN: 0-674-21673-3.

34. Reichgott M. Lecture: the impaired physician: focus on substance abuse. Alchohol: Albert Einstein College of Medicine; 2005.

35. Crowley TJ. Doctors abuse reduced during contingency-contracting treatment. Alcohol Drug Res 1985–1986;6:299–307.

36. Terry K. Impaired physicians: speak no evil? Med Econ 2002;79(19):110–2.

Index

Note: Page numbers of article titles are in **boldface** type.

Oral Maxillofacial Surg Clin N Am 22 (2010) 537–540
doi:10.1016/S1042-3699(10)00114-7
1042-3699/10/$ — see front matter © 2010 Elsevier Inc. All rights reserved.

oralmaxsurgery.theclinics.com